HARVEST MOON

SALLIE TISDALE

HARVEST MOON

Portrait of a Nursing Home

HENRY HOLT AND COMPANY
NEW YORK

Published by Henry Holt and Company, Inc.,
521 Fifth Avenue, New York, New York 10175.
Published in Canada by Fitzhenry & Whiteside Limited,
195 Allstate Parkway, Markham, Ontario L3R 4T8.

Library of Congress Cataloging in Publication Data
Tisdale, Sallie.
Harvest Moon.
Bibliography: p.
1. Nursing homes—United States.   2. Nursing home
care—United States.   3. Nursing home patients—United
States.   I. Title.
RA997.T57   1987   362.1'6'0973   87-25
ISBN: 0-8050-0565-X

First Edition

Designed by Kate Nichols
Printed in the United States of America
1   3   5   7   9   10   8   6   4   2

ISBN 0-8050-0565-X

For the memory
of Barbara Myerhoff

Acknowledgments

This book would not exist except for the gracious cooperation of the people who live and work in the nursing home I have chosen to call Harvest Moon. I have given them pseudonyms to protect their privacy, but that is all: the incidents and conversations I record are real.

This work has been favored by the attention of a meticulous editor, Channa Taub, who seemed to understand and clarify my ideas before I did. I am very grateful for her efforts, and for the help and support offered by my agent, Katinka Matson.

I would like to thank Art Kleiner, for friendship and editing; Linda Duggan for her comments and our sorority in nursing; and John and Margery Benson, readers, nurses, and abiding friends.

Marcella Gauthier helped type and showed me which buttons to push on the keyboard.

My husband, Bob Macer, has given me so much in time, patience, and ideas; all I do is partly his.

This book is dedicated to Barbara Myerhoff, the author of *Number Our Days* and other works of personal anthropology, for what has to be called a pioneering attempt to combine the subjective experience with objective observations. I wish she could read my own effort.

Shine on, shine on harvest moon,
Up in the sky—
I ain't had no loving since
January, February, June or July.

Introduction

Florence taught me to sing, not well, and we would sing and skip and laugh out loud. I knew her years ago, in my first job in a nursing home. I was a nurse's aide, I was seventeen, and she was in her seventies. Florence was confused, happily so, unsure from moment to moment of her age, her history, her condition and status in life. She was not inclined to wonder, happy to accept whatever explanations I and others would offer for the apparent inconsistencies in her life. She sang a few songs many times: "I ain't had no loving since January, February, June or July!" And skipped a step on her walk to the dining room.

One afternoon she beckoned me over to her room, where she waited in the doorway. She leaned over close to me to whisper in my ear, pointing surreptitiously to her roommate, an obese and balding woman sleeping in a chair by the window. "That woman," Florence told me, enunciating carefully. "She told me her family put her in a *nursing home*." She widened her eyes in proper shock at such a thing. "Can you imagine? Isn't that *awful?*"

And oh, yes, Florence, I wanted to say. Oh, it is awful.

We all die, and most of us grow old, and for a certain inevitable number of us age brings its sisters: dependence, frailty, and a gut-wrenching perishability. Age is the last place and time most of us will inhabit, and the fact that age seems so foreign to most of us, as though cleft from the known world, is one of life's sly tricks. It is outside the compass points, outside the native land we dwell in till we reach it. The time comes, for most of us, when we have to consider—for ourselves or someone we love—those awful places, those terrible, necessary institutions, those nursing homes.

This terribleness is not always obvious. Ordinary, even familial things happen here, though often unwitnessed. Wounds are healed, muscles strengthened, faces washed, and hands held. Each small movement is tiny in its fruition, huge in its absence. But in spite of these gestures, to most people the nursing home remains a cockeyed slanting world, without common reference, begging despair. Finding no one to blame for old age, why not blame those who house it?

This despair—felt not only in the presence of such things but simply from the *knowledge* of such things—is both personal and organic. "I pray to God I die before this happens to me," murmurs the wife or the son, gazing sideways at the old and irrevocably dying relative. It is like an experience of others' pain giving life to one's own before it is felt. The death of other people, witnessed in slow, trivial steps, becomes the death of oneself, too soon. The queer conversation of the confused telegraphs one's own inevitable, terror-struck annihilation. All these losses are like giant secrets, or errors, in the machinery, that take place not with a dramatic excitement—it would be almost more bearable if they *were* accompanied by fireworks and lightning—but with a plodding, daily dullness.

I can see it all another way. The sameness of each day shaves away the apparent passage of time. It makes something different of time, something insignificant, until the day's routine is the simple facts of bodies, people, dependence, and the paring down of borders that hold us separate.

I like nursing homes. I have since I first took a job in one, and learned without knowing what I was really learning how to change a bed with a person in it—a very old, fragile, dying person who watched my every move from silent eyes. At seventeen I was struck with the intimate knowledge of age's force. I was too young to know how young I was, to know I should have thought of myself apart, separated, from the old people I tended. Without knowing what I was learning, I learned about age as though I, too, would grow old in the course of things. Old age, and the delicate, powdery skin, the brittle bones and coarse hair—the outward signs of an internal passage of time—quickly became normal, even ordinary things, and in a vital way unimportant.

This is our world, for better or worse. By their nature nursing homes are self-justified worlds, concerned with problems, crises, and solutions of no concern to the culture at large. They exist precisely because their concerns aren't shared by the culture at large—created to manage those unavoidable concerns abdicated by that same culture.

Standing apart this way, almost parenthetically removed from its environment, the nursing home becomes a kind of tribal village, a place of misfits. It has a language of its own, customs of its own. It is slightly out of plane, not quite polite, designed for people who have no other place to go, no other place to be, who don't mingle with the rest of us. Nursing homes are communities of people incapable of claiming more than they receive, utterly at the mercy of our goodwill. I have been in enough nursing homes for enough years to become a part, a participant in a world of unexplained noises and strange sights, odd appearances and mysterious events, which at their heart are the most mundane of things. Nursing homes hold all the force and drama of life and death and the movements between, made manifest in earthly banality. This is where I travel, this is my family, my culture, where I live. I guess I have become a kind of expatriate here, hoping for visitors.

So, I have written a kind of travel guide, a gentle introduction to a foreign land. I often felt curious about how the whole mechanism worked—how communities of 50, 100, 350 people worked together, with the added piquancy of long-term illness and need. What are the shifting relationships like? What is communicated, what forgotten? What are the little moments, tiny things, glimpsed from the side as though driven by at top speed, half-seen: Did I really see that? Did she really say that? All these things are mysteries, all familiar. I found a nursing home gracious enough to open its doors to me, and I watched. In the course of my months in Harvest Moon I found myself caught up not only in big concerns, in questions of considerable size, but in many small concerns, too—in a single step, and how to take it, a single bite of food, a glass of water, a snowfall, a memo, a glance.

I am still surprised by how much there is to see that I'd missed in my headlong rush of nursing, and how much I had to miss still because so much happens at once. What immensely detailed lives we lead, each of us, even in bed, even shuffling down a bare hall, even sleeping in a chair, dreamy, confused. This is a kind of picture, angle and line, gleam of light, shape, with empty spaces and shadowed corners. Pictures always have frames, and something outside them; stories always have silences, and this one is no exception.

HARVEST MOON

CHAPTER ONE

Harvest Moon

She is a little foreshortened now, her bones drawing slowly into themselves, taking up less space. But Anna Rosenbaum was always short. She grew up in the streets of Brooklyn, poor, tough, leading with her dramatically hooked nose. Anna came to San Francisco more than fifty years ago and worked as a waitress in all-night cafés and bars on Fisherman's Wharf.

Anna never married; she hints at bad affairs and back-street, window-breaking lovers' spats. She is an alcoholic, and has spent most of the last ten years in and out of welfare hotels, sleeping in the unkempt beds of other restless people, sleeping, sometimes, in doorways. Anna never stopped to imagine her future, which came too slowly to see, edging up behind her and fueled by long nights, hard drinking, and faithlessness.

Anna's hips, like other things, have failed her. One, porous and weak, was replaced surgically with a shiny promise of steel—a broken promise. The other hip became so badly infected that, in the end, the surgeons threw up their hands and cut the whole joint out. Her legs are different lengths now, twisted unnaturally sideways and back. In the last year, no longer able to walk, she has checked herself in and out of several nursing homes, playing each time the part of the perennial bad girl at parochial school—smoking in the elevators, climbing over the bedrails, disappearing for hours, and, always, mocking those around her with a stream of abuse.

Her cheeks hang loose and jowly from a dry, emaciated face. Her eyes bulge in exophthalmic surprise on either side of a nose broad and long as a bridge abutment. She has no teeth, won't wear dentures: her tongue is chronically inflamed. "My tongue's a mess, see?" she says, sticking out the swollen, yellowed muscle. "They tell me I got a bacteria. I can't urinate. I can't move my bowels. I'm crippled. It's a helluva way to live, I tell you."

Decades of smoking have coarsened and lowered her voice to a trembling tenor, still thick with Brooklyn. At night she sings to herself, old songs from earlier years, the ones that men in San Francisco bars would use for raucous serenades, before bursting into loud laughter. She entertains herself by deriding the nurses—"They kick me and I kick them"—and giving her jewels of wisdom to her visitors, who are all professionals, all social workers and their ilk. Her family is gone, her friends dead or lost.

Every day the physical therapists here strap a three-inch block of wood to her shorter leg, brace it around into a semblance of order, and help her to stand. She must make progress, must leave her wheelchair behind or her Medicare will be cut off. Today she insults the aide, shaking her head, then insults herself. She stands in the doorway of the therapy room, a little woman frowning in a crowd of well-wishers, and counts out loud to three before rising. The change is abrupt and complete. Her face falls into ruins and she cries.

"I can't do it, honey, I can't do it." Her legs tremble, she slides backward into the chair with strong hands guiding her. "Oh, honey, you get old too soon and smart too late."

Harvest Moon Care Center is a nursing home for one hundred people, located in a residential neighborhood in a medium-

2

sized West Coast city. The architecture is undistinguished, the landscaping ordinary and not quite finished. The walls inside are broad and painted in cheap, dull colors, decorated with amateurish oil paintings of fruit bowls and flower vases. In these characteristics Harvest Moon is like most of the thousands of nursing homes in the United States. In some respects, though, Harvest Moon is different, even unique. It is owned by a large fraternal organization with a long-standing interest in caring for the elderly, and has a good reputation in the community. People sometimes wait months for a vacancy here. In a market turning toward for-profit corporate control at an almost frantic pace, Harvest Moon remains decidedly nonprofit, surviving partly on donations and second-hand equipment, and run by a board of directors determined not to sink in an increasingly cutthroat market.

It is mid-October, a Tuesday, and at ten thirty in the morning the sky over Harvest Moon is still overcast and cold. I stand at the central core of four hallways by the long nurses' desk, called the station. Each of these hallways is populated by a shifting assortment of people and equipment. The walls are decorated with posters, two different kinds, all cartoons. One kind reminds workers to wash their hands; the other exhorts the reader to quit smoking. On the corner of one wall is a felt-penned sign with an arrow, saying CATHERINE'S ROOM THIS WAY. There are people walking, people riding in wheelchairs, people with canes, and they detour around tall shelves of empty, littered food trays, housekeepers' carts neatly stacked with white bottles of bleach and disinfectant, and cupboards with locked drawers full of medicine. An old woman sits on a high plastic chair with a hole cut out of the bottom. She is naked under the flannel sheet that wraps around her and cocoons her arms in against her body. Her withered feet and mottled, pale legs hang unprotected below the hem of the material. She stares ahead, unblinking, waiting to be showered. From behind a closed door comes a loud giggle. People break across the rock of the nurses' station, dispersing in every direction. In the odd corner created at the intersection, where the two halls don't quite meet, hangs a birdcage with a silent parakeet. Below the cage an old man in a wheelchair whistles a tuneless, wheezing song to the bird.

Paula Schulz is writing rapidly in a thick chart propped open on the chest-high counter at one end of the station. Paula is the nurse practitioner at Harvest Moon, a registered nurse with postgraduate training—in Paula's case, almost two years—in medical diagnosis and treatment. Paula is certified as a geriatric practitioner, specially trained in the care of the elderly. She works, nominally, under the supervision of Harvest Moon's medical director, a physician who visits briefly once every week or two. It is Paula's job to manage the medical care of the patients from day to day. She is a department of one, independent, moving through every department with equal dispatch. She wears red stretch pants over her full hips, a polka-dot red blouse with a big, silky bow tie, and a dark sweater. Over her clothes she wears a lab coat; its left breast is decorated with a half dozen medallions and pins of honor and association. She has short, dark, wavy hair flecked with gray, and bright dark eyes in a face both fit and attractive. On her wrist she wears a digital watch with a shiny vinyl band to match the red of her pants.

When Paula finishes her writing, she grabs an orange chart from a wall of files, each with a stripe of orange or blue or green, and strides quickly down the matching orange hall till she finds Phoebe White lying in bed. Phoebe White is ninety-one years old, a fine-boned, tall, white-haired woman with square glasses. She is pleasant, polite, almost patrician. She is confused, too, and struggles to explain the perplexity around her.

We had breakfast recently, Phoebe White and I, and I asked her if she would eat her eggs. "Are you going to eat your eggs?" I asked, pointing to the yellow mound in front of her. "Eggs?" she asked me, stalling, and I pointed again. "Well," she finally replied, pulling herself up, "I don't know what they are, so I'm not going to eat them." Across her face passed a kind of relief, at another obstacle conquered, another scene averted with minimum fuss.

Several days ago Phoebe fell into a slumber and wouldn't wake. She became feverish, and was taken to a local hospital for observation. The hospital released her a few days later, without an explanation, an I.V. needle stuck in her arm to provide fluids. Since that time she has refused to eat, and her weight has dropped. When the I.V. stopped working two days ago, she refused to allow another to be put in.

Paula asks her without preliminary if she has changed her mind about the I.V. Paula asks Phoebe every day; she is bound by law to offer food and water to every patient, every day. Phoebe smiles thinly with a trace of humor; she is sitting upright in bed and dressed in a flower-print housecoat. She has a delicate, almost vulnerable strength, like a long-dormant athlete. She looks capable of holding out for a long time.

"Don't you touch me," she answers Paula.

Paula is silent a moment, then smiles slyly herself, happily, and slowly reaches out with her index finger and pokes Phoebe in the arm. Phoebe sneers at her.

"*You* know what I mean."

Paula laughs and leaves, opening the chart as she passes out the door, already scribbling a note of the conversation.

Cathy Bosley, a plump blond woman in her late twenties who works as the activity assistant, heads briskly down the hall a half hour later. It is almost eleven and time for the weekly Trivial Pursuit game she conducts with a passion. As she passes Phoebe White's room she sees an aide helping Phoebe into a wheelchair; Phoebe, too, has a passion for the game, when she remembers. Cathy stops at the central hallway beside a small woman in a wheelchair.

"Are you coming to Trivial Pursuit?" Cathy asks, leaning down, hugging her arms possessively around the woman's shoulders. She speaks in a loud, cheery voice. Verna Livingston looks up at her from a few inches away with a sour face.

"All right, all right, I'll go," she finally answers. "You go first, then I'll go. All right, all right." She starts to turn the chair toward the dining room where the game is played. "I don't have anything else to do."

The dining room borders the double front doors, which in turn open to a crowded parking lot bordered with a hedge. Visitors enter the front hallway beneath a windblown American flag, pass a receptionist at a desk, and face the smokers' table in the dining room a few yards away, before they turn. Near this table a small quiet group gathers.

A sullen man in a white uniform positions the many wheelchairs in place at the table. When Phoebe White arrives she beams happily as she is parked beside Max Kleiner, a white-haired, lump-faced man with jug ears that pitch wildly out from his head. Since a stroke several years ago he has been unable to walk. Max talks in a stream of diphthongs and phonemes repeated in happy verbosity. Now he sits at the table laughing continually, head turning rapidly from face to face, following the movements of each person in the room.

"Wee-wee-wee, bay-bay-bay!" he cries. "Woo-woo, wee-wee-wee." Each phrase is uttered with maximum expression, the sounds of an infant discovering his toes, sounds of delight and invention, lewd in their insinuation of sensual promise. Max Kleiner's fat vowels are so close to actual words that listeners strain to understand until, with reflection, they finally turn to something else.

Phoebe turns to Max now and her face brightens with memory.

"That's him! That's the man! They had me married to him this morning!" she cries to the table, pointing to Max with a long finger. Then she turns to Verna Livingston beside her. "I'm Bernice's sister. She owns this place."

The sullen young man announces that the players should

separate the tiles in front of them into piles, and leaves the room.

"Why separate them?" asks Phoebe.

Verna answers, still sour. "I don't know. I don't know why."

"It doesn't make sense."

"No, it doesn't make sense."

"What's the point?"

"I don't know the point," says Verna, and reaches for a mound of tiles, beginning to stack them. Max reaches, too, but the aide has placed the tiles out of his grasp. He plays with his hands.

"If they're going to give us tea, I have a cookie," announces Verna. She holds up a pink napkin she has kept hidden in her lap. "Here's my cookie. I have one cookie and it's cracked."

Cathy Bosley, meanwhile, has pulled a stack of cards out of the Trivial Pursuit box and is ready to begin. The game requires only that Cathy read the question to the group. Whoever knows the answer calls it out. The first correct answer wins the speaker a tile, and when one person has collected three tiles, they are gathered back and the game begins again.

"Who was the 1960 *Sports Illustrated* Sportsman of the Year?" Cathy asks, speaking in a loud, ringingly cheerful voice. She glances around the table, then repeats the question.

"Bobby Orr." The voice belongs to Maude Davis, a ninety-three-year-old woman who rarely attends activities, preferring in her irritation the solitude of slow prowls and her room.

"That's right! Goodness, that's correct!" cries Cathy, shaking her head. She hands Maude a tile and Maude retreats into silence.

"Buddy, are they going to give us tea?" says Verna loudly. "I have a cookie."

"No," replies a husky, dark-haired young man down the table.

"Well, I guess I won't get to have my cookie, then."

"Who was Sherlock Holmes's smarter brother?" calls out Cathy. No one answers. Two nurse's aides walk in and head for the vending machines in the corner. Smoke drifts to the table from the three patients sharing a newspaper and smoking break nearby. Overhead four electric fans turn in lazy imitation of the slow pace below. Cathy repeats the question.

"Um, um, eighteen, um, eighteen seventy-nine!" says a woman hunched down in her seat.

Phoebe suddenly grabs Max's hand and smiles hugely; Max starts babbling with excitement. "Whoo-whoo!" he cries like a train whistle. "Whoo-whoo, ha-ha-ha, whoo-whee!"

Phoebe laughs happily. "Ouch! Ouch!" she giggles.

And this is how the days go, in dreamy conversations of unclear intent, jokes without punchlines, sorrows without end. The patients who retain their wits often avoid these gatherings, the odd meetings in the hallways, the chaotic winds of damaged cerebrums as much as possible. But they are here, too, and sometimes here to stay.

Here there is a constant going on, and a constant staying the same. Phoebe and Max and Verna lead lives of sameness disturbed by tiny and constant stimulations of brain and body. When I am in their midst it seems a world in continual refinement, even renewal. It is as though each member were almost, but not wholly, complete, and sought through the repeated, inactive days a final harmony, a topping off. Someday it will be my turn—to be old, to be sick, to feel my own dying surround me in a cloud of soft certainty. Perhaps someday I'll rock myself to sleep like Anna, singing old songs creakily in the dark, and the young face that passes briefly over mine like a revenant will pay no heed, bear no mind to the meaning of the words. It won't be that young girl's fault; she'll be too young to know.

A hum of activity underlies the passiveness—it is velocity without motion. It is, after all, a community of human beings going about their complicated and inexplicable business. But the climax is never reached. A Greek chorus murmurs in the background, and now and again individuals step forward, as though on cue, and deliver brief and poignant lines. These are the questions no one else thinks to frame.

Gertrude Werner is wearing a shiny pink raincoat, made of a nylon material that glistens in the fluorescent light as though already wet. Her hair falls lankly below her stooped shoulders. A nose flares out of her bony face, deepening her already sunken eyes. She steps up to the counter like a Fate, her stockinged legs peering out of the raincoat into pink slippers. She addresses the nurse on the other side.

"I heard you might have some scissors for sale," she says in a nasal German accent, politely, without hope.

"No, I don't," answers Bonnie Pereira, without looking up from the mound of paper in front of her. She gives the rapid response of one who has answered the same question before, a litany in unconscious memory.

"I didn't think you would," replies Gertrude, disappointed, unsurprised. She waits a moment, blankly, and just as she turns to go her face takes on a brief glow of animation. She turns back and manages to catch Bonnie's attention one more time.

"Yes?" asks Bonnie, weary, amidst the PA announcements and ringing phones and conversations that swim around her.

With hope now, with a slight concern, even with mild wonder, Gertrude leans over the counter and asks, "Do you know enough about why I'm here to tell me?"

CHAPTER TWO

Village Life

Harvest Moon has one hundred "beds," or room for a total of one hundred patients. Of these, sixty are set aside for "intermediate care," or the kind of basic nursing most often associated with nursing homes. Intermediate-care patients are not acutely ill, and not dying—at least, not of anything except age—but neither are they able to live independently. A few generations ago these patients would have been cared for in the back bedroom of the farmhouse, ministered to by women of various ages and degrees of relation, until their invalid state finally killed them. For some, like Max Kleiner and Phoebe White, their dependence is born of a combination of mental confusion and physical frailty. For others, brain-damaged young people like Buddy Mullin, even an abbreviated kind of independence would require a live-in aide, a remodeled home, equipment, and more. Intermediate-care patients are here, usually, for the long haul, for a stay of indeterminate length—months, and years, and often till death. They fill B Wing, painted blue, and D Wing, painted green, which face each other across the lap of the nurses' station. There are more than 1.2 million such patients in homes like this across the United States.

The third hall, C Wing, is a sickly orange, and has room for forty patients requiring professional nursing, or "skilled care." Ten years ago—for some, only a year or two ago—these patients would never have left the hospital. But a great number of people who used to spend weeks in the hospital didn't make use of many of the services provided—they used only the nurses, and sometimes therapists. Hospitals provide intensive care, which requires high technology, sterile and careful conditions for surgery, complex laboratories, and a morgue. But most hospital patients, after their initial crises, after their medical questions are mostly answered, just need nursing care. The hospital is too much, too big, too costly. Changes in Medicare law and simple economic necessity have created a new kind of nursing home care, and Harvest Moon was one of the first facilities in its area to open a wing for skilled nursing. The facility is run on a philosophy of "total rehabilitation," with therapy and its purpose—to enhance the quality of life, to improve each patient to their greatest possible level of functioning—available to every patient. Traditionally, rehabilitation has been considered the province of the healthier patients, the ones who may "get well," and those doomed to chronic illness were not given the opportunity to achieve such small and vital goals as feeding themselves, buttoning a shirt. This is still true to a large extent, again the product of economics as well as inflexible thinking. The staff of Harvest Moon has tried to overcome these set ideas, as much as money and time will allow, and remind each other in consistent small ways to see the possibilities dormant in each patient, however subtle. One result is a solid community reputation for good care, and a waiting list for intermediate-care beds.

The patients on C Wing are notable most of all for variety in condition and disease. Strokes, broken and repaired hips, and cancer make up the majority, but almost any illness can sooner or later be found there: uncontrolled diabetes, lung disease, infected wounds, comas, head injuries, heart attacks, and more. Skilled-care patients stay, ordinarily, for relatively brief spells—a few weeks to several months—before going home, returning to the hospital, being transferred to another nursing home providing more basic care (called an ICF, for intermediate-care facility), or dying.

The last hallway, and the longest, forming the long pole of the cross, reaches from the front door to the nurses' desk, and contains the administration offices, the kitchen and dining room, and the rehabilitation department. It provides a full complement of therapy: physical, occupational, and speech. Most of the rehabilitation services are used by skilled-care patients, such as those recovering from a stroke. But they are available to any patient who requires them.

Today Harvest Moon has ninety-seven residents for its one hundred beds. Eighty percent of the residents are over seventy years of age, but the youngest is seventeen. Almost eighty-five percent of them are women, blessed with longer lives.

In the last month there have been forty-three new people admitted, and forty-four discharged. Four of these died. Of the others, released variously to hospitals, other nursing centers, or their own homes, nothing is known. This is a self-perpetuating community, and absence from the community invokes a kind of absence in the minds of the remaining members, who are concerned with life here, now, moment to moment and day to day. The missing are gone, and no longer a concern.

There are almost 24,000 nursing homes in the United States. More than 19,000 of these are run for profit, by corporations, tax syndicates, and individuals. Nursing homes house two million people at a cost of over $30 billion annually—about eight percent of all the dollars spent nationally on health care. The population of the United States is growing steadily older, and among people over sixty-five, the "very elderly" group over eighty-five is growing significantly faster than any other.

The nursing home industry is booming—new nursing homes are constantly being built, old nursing homes remodeled and expanded. Nearly one million full-time employees work in nursing homes—at a turnover rate of sixty percent annually. Most areas of the United States suffer a chronic shortage of nursing home beds, so that thousands of people who can no longer care properly for themselves at home, who have no one to care for them, must wait on long lists for a vacancy. The shift is undeniably and inexorably toward profit; two corporations that run nursing homes as a primary business are on the New York Stock Exchange now, and each buys new nursing homes almost weekly. The small, privately run—often family-owned—nursing home, called the "mom-and-pop" nursing home by insiders, is almost a thing of the past. And in all this excitement, nursing homes run constantly short of staff, especially nurses and nurse's aides, so that a situation made difficult by the demands of profit-oriented budgets is made worse by a shortage of help.

Insurance plans, which often pay all the cost of a hospital stay above a certain level, usually pay for no more than two weeks of skilled care in a nursing home—and very rarely for any intermediate or chronic care. Medicare pays most or all of the actual cost of skilled care—again, for a limited time—but it pays nothing for intermediate care. Traditionally, the bill is paid out of pocket, from savings or the sale of the family home and assets. At Harvest Moon a bed in a three-bed room, with a bathroom shared by six patients, costs about $55 a day. This includes meals and nursing care, but not medication, doctor's visits, or any kind of therapy or supplies. On the skilled-care wing the cost is closer to $80, and can go up depending on the complexity of the nursing care required. Such costs destroy a family's financial security very quickly, and there is usually no alternative to the welfare system. The social service establishment calls this process "impoverishment," the making of a new class of poor. And the welfare system, administered primarily by the state, can set rates as they see fit. Harvest Moon is paid about $42 a day for each of its intermediate-care welfare clients; on every such patient the home loses money every single day.

New Medicare regulations, encouraging hospitals to transfer patients to nursing homes as soon as possible, have added a fury of change and bewildering complexity to the nursing home field. Nurses must learn new skills as fast as possible, till they hold in their palms the entire tapestry of a metropolitan hospital. Nurses, too, are demanding more: more recognition, more respect and money and benefits. The budget, though, is as tight as it has ever been, and drawing silently tighter. For everyone involved it is a world of velocity, without motion.

Another day, new questions, new voices, but always a poignant familiarity. I like to think these things, these little rivulets of interaction occurring on the periphery, are efforts to explain, to illuminate. Sometimes I tell myself that the very obscurity of these layered relationships is an explanation of a kind.

Phoebe White, propelling herself in her wheelchair by scooting forward with her feet, is hurrying as fast as she can. "Sister! Sister!" she cries to Verna Livingston ahead of her. I push her to catch up, but when she sees Verna's face she does an exaggerated double-take and says, dismayed, "*That's* not the mother! What's, what's the name of, of the man?" She points around her, upset.

Verna looks at her with disdain and wheels slowly off in the opposite direction, down B Wing. Phoebe is visibly disturbed by the desertion.

"Come *on*, come *on!*" she pleads to Verna's back, and an aide, annoyed, takes hold of her chair from behind and pushes her toward the dining room, telling Phoebe, "She doesn't want to go that way." Phoebe, in tears, shakes her head.

"Yes, she does. Yes, she does."

And before Phoebe is safely down the hall—but after her tears are dry and the scene forgotten—another scene begins, a sibling squabble.

Gertrude Werner has begun to chastise Angela Gonzales, a silent, acquiescent woman, severely retarded. She has been in

Harvest Moon so long as to have taken on a kind of absence; uncomplaining, apparently comfortable, she is as present as a file cabinet or the scale. She has a hump in her back that bends her forward in a curve. Gertrude has somehow become convinced that Angela is a recalcitrant little boy with bad posture; she takes this act of defiance personally. When she finds her, she berates her. As an aide steps forward to intervene on Angela's behalf, Gertrude starts pushing and tugging on her shoulders.

"Come on, little boy," she implores. "Hold your head up!"

It is a bickering family, a family in which cousins speak only to each other, the aunts only to the sisters-in-law. A certain amount of misinformation is inevitable. Grudges simmer, rumors turn somehow to unmitigated fact, accusations creep quietly underfoot. Every family has its secrets, and its sororities; every family its own magnetic center. Harvest Moon is bottom-heavy with unskilled labor paid the lowest wages, overseen by a small group of well-educated, well-paid professionals.

Walking the halls, one sees almost a caricature of social delineation, a stew of race and age and education, culture and language, motive and intelligence. Almost all the darker faces belong to housekeepers and janitors and kitchen aides, who include in their ranks Filipinos, Hawaiians, blacks, and Vietnamese. Almost all of the management is white and over forty years of age. Lying in bed are housewives, plumbers, retired nurses, schoolteachers, a symphony violinist, a ham radio operator, and a pediatrician in his nineties who claims to have delivered over two thousand children and disliked each one of them personally. Every person's image of every other person, of each event, is so different as to be incongruent with any other. Each person has at least one goal at odds with that of another person. The parceling out of power is most uneven.

In this place people who are very different from one another come to see their similarities, and also to see the subtle differences in people assumed to be the same. It is possible, this way, to find one's *place* in the community, a proper place of the correct size and shape. To work in a nursing home with any kind of contentment requires a balancing of the needs of self and other, an ability to give without expecting gratitude. My contentment comes and goes, and often seems to disappear completely; I feel bitter and acerbic and snap at the people I pass, hurriedly, down the halls, weighted by work never done and events never explained. And then it returns as suddenly, lit by moments when I pass out of myself into a continuum without a beginning or an end, at last a member and not a watcher. The search for this contentment, unlike any other, and the clues along the way, I feel almost as a compulsion. It drives me back to sounds and smells that might, without association, be unpleasant, but which have become through the years the sounds and smells of home. Wherever I travel within the culture I am at ease.

I drive to the suburbs to visit a friend, a nurse, happily in charge of improving a nursing home with a well-deserved bad reputation. She is proud of her efforts and the results of her hard work, and I can see the signs, I know the symptoms of good nursing care. I have grown intimate, too, with wheelchairs, their boxy size and stubborn axles and short stature; with the texture of elderly skin, smooth and dry, and its subtle shades of color, all pastel. I recognize the chorus, the chant of monotoned voices drifting down like light snow, calling "help me, help me, nurse, nurse"—and I hear both the content, and the meaning.

This is one of the meanings of community: recognition. I recognize the shapes and sizes and smells, the intention, the language. I fit in, have a place, because of experience: I am part of it because I have been part of it. I belong, and that is a rare thing—and rarer still, I belong to a tribe of people both needing and giving, dependent and independent in turn. I feel glad that the place I have found is one filled with the unending, unfolding stages I have yet to enter. It is as though I have been privy to parts of my own future, and found a way to embrace it.

Nursing homes are terrible places, people murmur to me. Terrible places. I know what they mean—this going on, this repetition, this sense of *consignment*. It explains some of the surge in home health nursing. The advertisements for home health often play on the guilt that is the particular burden of families who find themselves played out, unable to continue caring for an elderly and ill family member; families who reluctantly begin searching for a nursing home. What kind of person puts her mother in a nursing home? How can a family condemn Grandpa to an institution?

Home health agencies emphasize the desirability of "keeping the family together," of "letting Grandma stay in her own home." A kind nurse can help carry the bittersweet burden. The choice to keep a frail or ill relative at home is sometimes the right one—but sometimes it is not, and it is this failure to admit the proper place of the nursing home that bothers me. We don't live in extended families; the home hearth is often empty. There are many factors at work in such a decision, and they aren't all emotional ones.

One of the foremost factors is expense, for Medicare and Medicaid, or welfare, rarely will pay for home health care. Neither will many insurance plans. Round-the-clock home nursing is often more expensive than a nursing home, depending on the patient's needs. But there are other factors, too, that make their presence felt soon enough—and after months or years these can become extremely painful.

The most obvious is exhaustion. Nursing is hard work, difficult work, and it goes on all day and all night long. Grown men are not babies, no matter what illness they suffer from, and months of lifting, bathing, and turning take their toll. Months of broken sleep and interrupted meals add up, too. And with a relative at home, there is no relief. Nurses are glad to go home at the end of the day, for all the affection they may feel for their charges. The son and daughter cannot go home, take a day off, freshen up, and come back lively. After a few weeks or months the bell is answered less quickly, the many small needs attended to more perfunctorily. Proximity has its rewards, and its price.

There are two sides to the terribleness of the nursing home: one is the fear that the patients are not well cared for, their needs not met. There are bad nursing homes out there, unfortunately, and I wouldn't put my own mother in a lot of facilities I've seen. But the most vehement arguments against bad nursing homes come from nursing home employees who fight this steep battle of bad press. It is not always obvious how well a nursing home cares for its residents, because so much of what can be seen—so much of what appears terrible, smells and sounds and looks terrible—is not the fact of the nursing home, but the fact of age and illness. A visitor may see only a restraint, and a small woman pressing pitifully against it; the nurse nearby sees the woman's confusion and weakness, the broken hip lying in wait past her next step. The visitor hears the cries for help and the ringing of bells, and senses neglect, laziness; the nurse finishes one task and moves to another, and another, making mental notes, and knowing all along that the cries for help often don't cease when help is given—the cries for help have an almost metaphorical place in the work being done. They are the work-songs in the field.

It is an imperfect design, but the nursing home—both conceptually and physically—is designed for dependence. It is, in its way, both economical and precise—and more. Many of the people who come here to work for brief spells, to pass time between other, more desirable jobs, find themselves unable to go. By joining the community they become party to a compulsive concern for the patients, a hunger to know *what happens* to them, to affect what happens. A lot of people call it love, without apology. I call it community, and membership. It is a most comfortable and touching familiarity, a gut recollection of an unremembered, not yet experienced past.

Paula Schulz, the nurse practitioner, has a feral quality, with frequent, bared-teeth smiles full of impatience. Her smiles have a warning buried in them, not too deeply. She is good-looking, powerful, ineluctably adult and ripe. Above her desk is a sign reading, "Thank you for holding your breath while I smoke," and under it she smokes without ceasing, waving the smoke away from her visitors expansively, talking, almost always talking, squinting her eyes to concentrate.

"There really isn't anything I'm afraid of," she says. "Fear isn't a part of my nature. Anxiety, concern, worry maybe, but not fear." She has a big, sudden laugh, a throaty tenor voice. "I was raised with a bunch of boys and a tough German father. He didn't teach us to be afraid of things. In fact, he taught us *not* to be afraid of things."

She barbs her conversation with provocative teasing and sharp banter, then professes surprise that the nurses she teases are intimidated by her style. But by the time she has expressed her surprise, it has changed to disdain, that they would allow themselves to be intimidated by anyone. I have known Paula Schulz for three years, and I have both admired and feared her for all that time. She has often hurt my feelings and the feelings of those around me with unexpected and thorny criticism, with impatience, with frustration at failed if well-intentioned effort. And I have wanted her to admire me, to *like* me, with all that same force of will. I sit opposite her in her large, windowless office near the central hallway, and find myself hoping for her approval—to my own chagrin, and her surprise.

In the first years of her marriage, twenty-six years ago, she worked as a night-shift aide in the only nursing home in her small Midwestern town. "It was an interesting job," she recalls, "because you did not only the laundry in the basement of this three-story building with bedridden patients on the third floor, you did the ironing and the mending and gave the insulin shot to the diabetic in the morning." When she and her husband and children moved to the West Coast she worked as a bartender, waitress, and grocery clerk, and then again as a

19

nurse's aide. One day in 1969 Paula saw a television commercial advertising a local community college nursing program. By then her three children were all in school, and she decided, almost impulsively, to enroll. She started in the practical nursing program, a one-year commitment, but before graduation re-enrolled in the longer registered nursing program. Ten years later she had a bachelor's degree, a master's degree, and certification as a geriatric nurse practitioner. She will begin her PhD, in urban studies, next year.

"I became a nurse as an adult," Paula points out, with slight derision. "I wasn't a quivering, scared, insecure teenager. I was thirty years old and had my family half-raised."

Paula wasn't long for the hospital. "I didn't like acute care. It was very good experience; it really prepared me for geriatrics. But I didn't like discharging people to—where? And with information about them that wasn't anywhere near correct. There was a night RN job that opened up in the place where I'd been an aide, and I thought, 'I'm going to go to work there as an *RN* and I'm really going to shape things up!' You have those kind of aspirations, you know. So they hired me on nights, and in the interim, the two-week period between being at the hospital and going there to work, the director of nursing service left. And they called me and offered me the position. They really needed somebody. So I said, 'All right, I'll try it, but I *don't* know what I'm doing, and we'll work this on a week-to-week basis. And if I'm not doing it as I should, you let me know, and keep trying to hire somebody!' " Paula laughs her big guffawing laugh, thick in the throat and deep, and keeps talking through her laughter. "I guess I was the DNS there for a year or so. It was a very bad facility and had lots of problems, and I was very green and didn't know how to handle things very well. I was practically trying to take care of all those patients by myself, so I left."

After a similar stint at a less desperate facility, Paula entered the nurse practitioner program at a nearby university.

When she graduated, seven years ago, she came to Harvest Moon. She is happy in the job: "I'm at the peak of my profession," she tells me. "I think the reason I stay here, first of all, is that there's a big difference between profit and non-profit organizations. Here, monies that are made that aren't budgeted to be spent are put back into the facility, to improve the facility, to improve the quality of patient care. In a profit-based facility the first thing that comes out is the profit. *Then* if there's any left it's put back in. The philosophy of this place, too, is exceptional—the rehabilitation concept. It's one of a kind, as far as I'm concerned."

Her husband owns and runs a small appliance repair business. For years Paula and their three children, now all young adults, worked weekends and evenings helping him with bookkeeping, cleanup, and other chores. Last year Paula quit. "I told him, 'I don't need to be working for you. I chose to be a nurse, and I didn't expect you to help me with my nursing job. *You* chose to have this business, now *you* run it.

"I was taught as a child that if you want something done right, you do it yourself," she continues. "I've gotten some feedback from some people—after a few *years!*—about how I impact them. They see me as inflexible. They see me as, I think, bossy. I *am* a bossy person, but I also think my role here enhances that. I totally intimidate the nurses, without intending to. I guess it's because I have certain expectations, and when they don't meet those expectations I let them know. Maybe my expectations are too high. I'm *stuck* with my personality, I can't help it, I've had it all these years!" She is laughing again.

"I've done new procedures here cold turkey, with everyone watching in terror. I'm not willing to make a mistake—so I do my homework. The technology of nursing has never scared me, never. I figure out, okay, what is this, what's it doing, where does it go, what's the worst thing that could happen, and how do I prevent that from happening? I'm not afraid to ask people, either, how things work—to figure out the resources and go ask them. I'm not afraid to say I don't know. That's why I'm not afraid of making a wrong decision—I never *make* a decision unless I know it's the right one." Paula's self-assurance can be daunting. She doesn't always realize the power with which she moves through the world around her. "When I first came here I had a hard time with all these resources—all these people who knew things that you could ask about! The first two years here I stepped on a lot of people's toes, because I was so used to nurses being all things to all people. I thought I knew more about physical therapy than the physical therapist. After all, I'd supervised it."

She has a gift for finding the sore places in a person. It makes her a superior diagnostician, fluid, unfettered by textbook expectations. She has a feral instinct to protect, too, and feels the heavy weight of her patients' pain. People are drawn to her: grieving guilty relatives who are searching for the way to ask a question find Paula phrasing it for them. Her peers at Harvest Moon approach her, sometimes, with the same caution they might use around a strange, seemingly unfriendly dog. Dogs can bite without warning.

Another change is at work in Harvest Moon: a few months ago the board of directors fired the impractical and popular administrator after a tenure of several years, and hired in his place an experienced, business-trained man intent on financial control. He plans to bring the non-profit home out of the red, and find in its trim shape a small profit to be recycled through again. One of his first acts was to cut the nursing staff.

Roger Scarpelli is a handsome, gray-haired man in his early fifties with a neatly grizzled salt-and-pepper beard. He dresses in smooth grays and slate blacks and an occasional pastel for a touch of the unique. He doesn't knot his ties, but folds them over as though still on a hanger. Roger Scarpelli has a deceptively soft, almost slurring voice; his speech is warm and friendly and sprinkled with small, ingenuously self-deprecating remarks. His tone has, too, a deliberate dignity, the straight posture of someone who knows they tend to slump. His slaps on the shoulder are jovial and filled with iron.

He is the new administrator of Harvest Moon. He says, unself-consciously, that he likes his position because "it gives me a chance to serve mankind in an area most people don't even like to think about." He is given to words like *humanitarian* and *service*. His syntax and vocabulary seem the product of too many seminars in management techniques; watching him run a meeting, you can see the conscious strokes he offers his employees. He uses verbs like *dialogue* and *input*, with a deceptive fellowship. When he disagrees with something he says, "I have a difficult time with that."

In free moments he walks down the hallway and times how long it takes for call bells to be answered by the nurses. The longest time he has recorded—he uses a second hand—was two minutes and fifteen seconds. "That is too long," he says. He assumes visitors make the same spot checks. "I wait and I look at my watch and pretty soon someone will come out of a room, and they're hurrying," he says. "They're busy, I know." He is wistful. He hopes for better times.

Scarpelli worked in manufacturing when he first finished college, then ran a small business which he soon sold for a tidy profit. Then he "laid around for a while. That was a nice time," he recalls. "I got to walk my daughter to school every day. There's a lot to be said for being comfortable in your middle age, and I got to be with my family." When he began to look for a challenge, a friend in hospital administration told him to try long-term care. Scarpelli took the bait. He was hired by a profit-based corporation to improve newly acquired homes, and after several years took on a major renovation. When the facility he helped turn from a run-down nursing home into a full-scale, multiservice care center was sold, he was fired by the new owners. "I expected that," he says. "They bring in their own people. It's part of the game."

His predecessor at Harvest Moon was named Art Kleaver. "Art was not a manager—I don't know what Art was," says Barbie Moscowitz, the dietician. "He was a wonderful guy. He needed a lot from people and people knew they could always get a lot from him. He was an aesthetic type, very bright, but not very down to earth." Kleaver developed education programs, panel discussions, and open houses. He expanded rapidly and encouraged more staff, more advertising. But he couldn't balance the budget. Roger Scarpelli, on the other hand, says his main purpose is to inspire an "efficient response" from the people he supervises.

Hundreds of thousands of dollars go in and out of Harvest Moon every month. Scarpelli says that salary and benefits are over eighty percent of his costs. Everything from long-term loan payments to new equipment and building repair comes from the remainder. Until the last quarter, Scarpelli's second as administrator, Harvest Moon had lost money—had lost money for ten years, a percent at a time. This time, the books show a half-percent profit.

Not everyone appreciates either Scarpelli's mission or his style. One nurse's aide says simply, caustically, "He's king, and he rules." Scarpelli confesses to an urge to be the "Lee Iacocca of long-term care," to move higher up in administration, to work at a corporate level, always, he adds, with the desire to serve as "the bottom line. That's why I have something to prove here with my management style." He brushes aside the accusation that he cut staff, preferring instead to call it "consolidation."

Every Friday morning at nine Roger meets with what he likes to call the "key personnel": the department heads, including Janet Krause, the director of nursing; Barbie Moscowitz, the dietician; Nancy Rice, the social worker; and Edie Douglas, his administrative assistant, who manages the budgets and policies for nursing and rehabilitation. Edie is Janet's direct supervisor; it is a friendly relationship.

Janet Krause arrives before Roger today. As she walks into the room she says, with the mild command typical to her voice, "Mrs. Weller fell. She's getting X rays now." Janet looks at Edie Douglas. "She had no orders for restraints." The room, and Edie, accept in silence.

Roger arrives and immediately moves to the head of the table in the small room filled almost entirely by a large table and several chairs. Barbie Moscowitz lays out a coffeepot and Styrofoam cups, critically testing the heat of the water before pouring. As Roger shuffles his papers, smiling and chatting, Edie, a fastidiously dressed woman in her fifties, reaches up to the thermostat and turns it to seventy. Roger buries his face in his hands. "Oh!" he moans loudly. "It's not *cold!*" Edie laughs, and scurries back to her chair.

Roger begins with a discussion of the emergency telephone list, long out of date and disorganized. He asks that an electrician, plumber, and furnace repairman who will take night calls be put on the list. He'd also like to try a rotating on-call plan for emergencies, to spare the uneven burden they put on the nursing department. Most emergencies happen on nights and weekends—it is often this inconvenient timing that makes them emergencies. At such times the nurses are the only staff in the building, except for a skeleton crew of housekeepers, perhaps a janitor. The nurses, faced with a blown electrical circuit or flooding bathroom, call not the head of maintenance or the on-call fix-it shop, but their boss: Janet Krause. "They call me because they know me," says Janet. "I'm not going to hang up on them." She is weary of the calls that come almost every night.

Roger finds only shallow support for his plan. Much as the other department heads sympathize with Janet, they feel little interest in taking their turn. Each feels he or she puts in time and effort beyond the call of duty already. They would rather take their chances on the old system: a list of phone numbers, unordered, for the nurses to choose from. He sighs, determined, and then says, "We're gonna do it *my* way, and *you're* gonna instruct your departments on how to do it right. I want you to think about it next week, so we can go ahead and dialogue on it later."

After half an hour, Edie gets up quietly and turns down the thermostat, and Roger looks up from his papers dramatically. "*Thank* you!" he breathes, rolling his eyes, and everyone laughs.

The maintenance supervisor mentions that there have been staff complaints about how poor the outside lighting is on the night shift. Several people are unsurprised; others, including Janet Krause, are slightly shocked. "There's no *light?*" she asks. "You mean when the nurses come to work in the evening they have to walk through the parking lot in the dark?" The explanation is simple. Each bulb for the large spotlights costs about $80, and they are notoriously fragile. The maintenance supervisor agrees to look for alternatives, and Roger agrees to find the money, from somewhere, to buy the bulbs.

Before the meeting ends, Edie Douglas mentions that odors are a problem again, after improving for a time. Smells of kitchen steam and urine, mop buckets and laundry, disinfectant and feces mingle together in the halls. Constant vigilance is not enough. "It's the kind of person we have here, too," adds Roger. "The dying. It has its own smell. I have to give credit to the girls for going in the room sometimes." The discussion drifts a bit, to long-gone patients, to patients soon gone, then Roger Scarpelli pulls it back, slowing the conversation, to close. "Let's keep dialoguing it back and forth," he finishes, and the meeting is over.

Paula Schulz remembers almost every patient she has known in seven years at Harvest Moon. They are, after all, hers in a way few people can become the property of another person—through the memory of skin and powerlessness, a kindness offered without return. She loves them in all her pragmatic busyness. I understand; I read the obituaries every day, seeking

26

the names of people I might have known for only a few days, never to see again. And when I find a familiar name, I feel a bit of pleasure at the nostalgia, in the very moment I feel sadness that now I will, truly, never see them again.

It is a measure of the familial, as well as the very long infirmities borne by some, that I recognize people when I come to Harvest Moon, patients I have cared for in other places, other buildings. Anna Rosenbaum is one; I saw her face, proud, ugly, and a little frightened, and knew her without hesitation. I had cared for her months earlier in another place, until she signed a release and left one day, unannounced. The first day we met I helped her sign for a Social Security check; making conversation, I asked her how she planned to spend it. She melted me with scorn. "Why, honey," she said, rasping through a cigarette, "I'm going to get drunk, what else?"

There are others who remain rooted in my mind, frozen at the moment I last saw them—leaving work, waving good-bye, already distracted by other things, errands, babysitters. They are moved by family or condition or act of God and the body to another place, another form; so many hundreds of people passing briefly under my hand—a body washed, a back touched or mouth cleansed, and then gone. I am unreasonably happy, then, to see on the wall of files at Harvest Moon a few familiar names. No illusion, they won't remember me—but to duck my head in a door and see again a face in memory is a fine thing.

Laura Lembke is falling off the pillow—the big, fluffy, white-cased pillow her devoted daughter gave her. She is falling sideways, one eye closed, the other half-open. Her hospital gown is crooked, exposing a soft, fat shoulder, and her thin, dry white hair flies around her head like a crown. She is round, squat, and all her parts are the same: small, perfectly round, apple eyes in a round, pink, powdery face. She looks like a snow creature shaped by careful, dreaming children. Her right hand holds a delicate Japanese fan. Her little pink mouth is dusted with food stains.

I lean over her bed. "Laura? Laura, are you all right?" She looks quite dead, but when I say her name louder her eyes flicker.

Laura tells her daughter, who visits every day, long stories—that she has won the lottery, that the "nice people" who work here take her out to dinner every night. One employee calls her Scarlett O'Hara.

"Are you all right, Laura?" I call, even louder, and then she wakens, exactly the woman she was six months ago, twelve months ago, a little surprised, as though she'd suddenly had the breath knocked out of her. Her voice, when she answers, is wispy and slightly whining, a child's voice, and very soft.

"Oh, I'm fine, dear," she says slowly, so that it's clear she is not, and the arm slowly rises until she can begin fanning herself. She still lies sideways between the bedrail and the pillow, watching me. She is a five-year-old girl in dress-up clothes: today she is pretending to be a sick old woman and this, she imagines, is how a sick old woman acts. She retains a remarkable sense of the melodramatic. I help her upright and soon leave, her attention wandering to the window, the fan slowly beating a breeze across her cheek.

On the way out of her room I see Cecil Lunt, restrained in a wheelchair by a broad mesh vest tied behind him. He is well over six feet tall, and was gaunt when I first met him more than three years ago, a diabetic with heart problems and Alzheimer's disease, his health rapidly failing because his confusion interfered with his medical care. He would not eat, would not take medication, instead gritting his teeth implacably against such intrusions. He careened down the halls, striding perilously and headlong across the floor, zigzag, rushing. We let him wander until he started to fall. As the disease worsened so did his behavior, deteriorating into biting, hitting, kicking, fits of yelling.

Today he is, surprisingly, still alive, shuffling his feet, bonier, thinner than ever, silent. His mouth is open in an expression of perpetual disbelief, his scalp is utterly bare, shiny, mottled with age spots. When the nurse arrives with his medicine he drinks it without protest. I touch his hand, his arm, call his name, and he doesn't respond. He stares ahead, shuffling his feet and going nowhere but on and on, never moving when I straighten up and walk away.

Is it all just unbearably sad, dreary, *wrong* somehow to find pleasure of a kind in such scenes? I am not supposed to, I know; my dark jokes, the laughter, is sometimes viewed with a slightly horrified scorn. It would be better to be grim, to settle for a bleak despair beside Cecil Lunt, an embarrassed blush for Laura Lembke. How can I explain the gratification, the sense of a hunger fed by such simple contacts? I need the absurdity, the quirks as much as the caring; they provide the balance so essential. It works for me in part because of compassion—not sympathy, not empathy—but something made of equal parts love and disinterest. The love is nothing distant, either, nor academic, but love born of experience, sweaty in the embrace of the real and immediate. It is made bearable by dispassion. To do otherwise is to love another's pain, for the pleasure of not feeling it. I am learning to love and be present in the face of whom I love without interest, without an agenda of what I need or expect from that moment of contact. I am learning to love disinterestedly. Disinterest is a kind of respect—a recognition of another person, separate and complete, and not so very different. I cannot forget them, so nearly newborn, cannot stop following their trembling course through an unforgiving, shortsighted world. Brief conversations that never conclude, small moments suspended—these are the only rewards to be found. And they are great, precious, gleaming jewels of satisfaction that take me out of myself and into a blurred world where age and youth are the same.

CHAPTER THREE

Teamwork

On October 20, Viola Cook died. On October 27, Gus Romano died. On October 29, Regina Brewster died. On November 5, two days ago, three patients died within hours of each other. One of them, Wendell Porter, had been in Harvest Moon for less than twenty-four hours. For several days beforehand the memo listing the expected day's admissions had contained his name, but each day a second memo had canceled his arrival. Each day the hospital discharging him decided his condition was too "unstable," until at last he was hurried over in an ambulance to Harvest Moon.

Another person who died that day, Patty Willett, was a blind woman in her fifties with ovarian cancer. She spent her days telling her visitors and nurses about the ham radio work she had done for decades. "She had friends all over the world," says Bonnie Pereira. "She took a *long* time to die. We would come in every morning and say, 'Patty Willett's *still* here?' "

Harvest Moon averages one death a week, and three admissions and discharges every two days—but nothing occurs on the average. The deaths, like the comings and goings of the living, arrive in handfuls, bound together like a nosegay. Each change in status, as it were, requires a machinery of paperwork and communication; newly admitted patients must be examined, discussed, dressed, unpacked, and greeted in certain ways. Something of the reverse happens when patients leave: they are discussed, packed, dressed, given packets of paper and medicine to pass to the new caregiver, or, occasionally, to take home. And when patients die, they too must be examined and dressed and packed; discussions of some kind, with some relation or official, must take place, and a sheaf of papers and medicine (and dentures, glasses, shoes, pajamas, and more) is given them to carry away.

Soon after a person's arrival, a "care plan" is prepared for the individual. It is a written set of goals and plans that reflects the efforts of the "care team"—the staff in nursing, medicine, therapy, and social work. The simple moments of care take place beside the bed, kneeling by a chair, while people sleep. The industry of care—the complicated enterprise of commerce, labor, and budget that fuels the simpler moments—is defined by certain words, frequently repeated, and by certain forms, frequently filed. The capacious pile of paperwork is the visible product of an endless cycle of meetings, formal and informal, of phone calls, regulation books, research, and the more subtle changes of social pressure and philosophical sophistication. The often-mutant evolution of Medicare and state health regulations must be second-guessed: a way, however narrow, must be found through the maze.

Medicare and other "third party payors"—insurance and welfare—require not only that the care given be recorded in certain ways at certain times by certain people, but that the care be justified on a daily basis. The payors like particular words and phrases better than others, words which have come to represent by abbreviation time spent and effort made. Turns of phrase colored by the fashion of changing mores, they reduce to a workable size and comfortable anonymity the patients and the staff.

Every Monday and Thursday the care team of Harvest Moon meets for lunch in the small front conference room tucked away across the hall from the receptionist. Lunch is brown bag and vending machine; the conference begins promptly at noon and lasts one carefully timed hour. Paula Schulz, the nurse practitioner, runs these meetings; she begins when her watch reads twelve o'clock, whether or not people are seated—or even present. Every newly admitted patient is reviewed within a week of admission, and a care plan is written; new patients are reviewed several times in the following few months. Patients whose care is being covered by Medicare are reviewed every *week* for the first month of their stay. Other stable and long-term patients are reviewed at least once a quarter. Paula Schulz keeps a rotating list of who is due for review; the team members are expected to come prepared with brief summaries on the status of each person due that day. They speak in a preordained order, rapidly, reading notes aloud, and take turns writing the agreed-upon catchwords in the chart. A kind of regulated brainstorm is at work, time-honored, unmolested, week after week after week.

Sometimes it works and sometimes it fails. When Margery Todd, the activity director, asked for help in finding ways to work with an elderly Japanese Buddhist, the best the team could come up with was to offer her soy sauce with meals. There are "typical" patients—with uncomplicated strokes or fractured hips—who follow expected patterns and present no unusual problems. Even terminally ill and comatose patients often fall into familiar categories, and can be swiftly dealt with by the use of proven methods. The written goals reek of therapeutics: "maximize level of function" is a very common one. Paula remarks as she writes for such a patient, "It sounds like a terminal diagnosis."

Promptly at noon, Paula pulls the first chart from the multicolored pile in front of her. "Buddy Mullin," she reads, "twenty-five-year-old male patient of Dr. Strand, hypoxic brain injury due to motor vehicle accident, cognitive defects." She reads without expression, rapidly, as she has read these phrases many times before. Buddy has been a resident of Harvest Moon for over four years, since soon after the car accident that left him with extensive and permanent brain damage. In that time he has learned to walk again—in halting, crude steps behind a walker, half the length of the hall twice a day. He has learned to talk again, in short, staccato bursts of speech. He has learned a sureness of himself, too, so that in the sweet, accidental naïveté of his damaged brain, he is happy to wear his hair in sleek black curls like Michael Jackson, to squeeze my hand, when I offer it, as hard as he can to show me his strength. He has made of this place a family. His own relatives no longer visit him. His bills are paid by welfare.

Nancy Rice, the social worker, takes time in the lackadaisical discussion to remind everyone that he continues to progress. She is tall and soft-spoken, and talks with a Southern murmur.

"He could end up in a foster home one of these days," she says.

"He's thirteen, he'll always be thirteen," replies Paula in disagreement.

Nancy shakes her head. "But I remember when he was ten. If you don't watch out, I may have to start looking for another placement for him, and I don't have the time."

Finding new "placements"—other places to live—for patients is one of Nancy Rice's main responsibilities. She is in charge not only of helping families cope with the worries and concerns, both financial and emotional, of having their relative in a nursing home, but of planning—sometimes from the day of admission—that relative's eventual discharge. Since Harvest Moon is well-known in the community and often has no room in its intermediate-care wings, Nancy frequently must find an intermediate-care bed elsewhere for patients who no longer qualify for Harvest Moon's skilled wing. There are lower levels of care than intermediate, too: some patients, those who can walk short distances and help a little with their personal care, feed themselves and use a toilet without too many accidents, might qualify for a retirement home. The community has a number of small, privately run foster homes, too. Foster care is often provided in a private home licensed by the state to care for elderly or dependent adults: the managers and staff are occasionally nurses, more often aides or simply individuals who go into the business the way private day-care providers go into the business of baby-sitting. Adult foster care typically provides shelter, meals, laundry, and some personal care, with twenty-four-hour supervision of some kind for people who cannot live alone. Although state and federal programs—mainly SSI, or Supplemental Security Income—pay a substantial portion of the costs of adult foster care and other "board and care" facilities like retirement homes, no federal agency collects data on them. It is literally unknown how many people live in such places, or whether the proper care is always provided. When Nancy Rice goes looking for a foster home, she has to dig deeply to be sure she has found the right place. It is this change to a more homelike atmosphere that Nancy imagines she may one day offer Buddy, a chance to live in a home setting with other disabled adults, under the watchful eye of an aide or nurse—a chance to be with people his own age, with a room of his own. She smiles at the thought. He would be sorely missed.

A female patient has been running away. It is she who is supposed to follow the arrowed signs, pointing out CATHERINE'S ROOM. She disappeared five times in one evening last week, and was found once sitting in the dumbwaiter to the laundry room. Nancy makes a note to seek a better placement for her as soon as possible, preferably a "secure"—that is, locked—wing in a facility equipped for such confused and mobile patients.

Maude Davis, the patient with unexpected prowess in Trivial Pursuit, is next. She has become quite famous, in her tenure of several years, for unfocused hostility and sudden obscenities. Her moods are unpredictable, capricious. She often refuses company of any kind, being weak only to the charms of Willie, the fat Hawaiian man who washes dishes and wheedles her attention with kitchen treats.

"She's generally happier talking to the figments of her imagination than she is talking with us," says Margery Todd, the activity director, who tries to visit every patient once a week. She is soft, fat, maternal; her almond eyes are outlined in black. "The goal here is improved socialization," she adds, pointing to her papers. "It's never going to happen, but we have to try."

"She responds *very* well to men," says Paula with a lascivious smile.

"Not to me, she doesn't," says Martin King, the physical therapist and the only man in the room.

"She let me do a vaginal exam on her once," Paula adds irrelevantly. "I was kind of hoping she wouldn't!" She laughs loudly.

"Paula Schulz, where's your professionalism?" Janet Krause, the director of nursing, is only half kidding.

Paula puts aside the chart and picks up the last one. She is suddenly serious.

"Rebecca Franks. She's not due for review. I'm asking this as a special request of the team because I think we can do something with her now. Correct that—I think we *have* to do something with her now."

Paula quickly summarizes the history: Mrs. Franks was admitted a few months before to a retirement home, a move she had not wanted to make. On her first day there she fell and severely broke a hip. She was bedridden for over two months and, from the beginning of her hospitalization, was confused. Paula is convinced that the confusion is related to the bad situation—the move, the injury, the surgery and recovery. Her physicians assume she is simply senile, and have given no orders for any therapy or treatment.

"I want a super-massive effort to bring her back to some

kind of independence. The family is fairly together about this. But no one wants to pay for it." Without physician's orders, Medicare will not cover therapy. She is not eligible for welfare, and the family cannot afford it. Rebecca Franks is alert, noisy, refuses to walk or feed herself, and has already crawled over her bedrails once and fallen again. She seems an unlikely candidate for a quick return to normal.

Paula looks pointedly at Charlene Parrott, the slightly disheveled, blond occupational therapist. "Charlene told me this is a real long shot. She's out in the ozone. But I said, 'You know me, Charlene, always betting on the long shot!' "

Charlene laughs, a barking sound. "Yeah. She thinks she's forty-six years old, single, healthy, doesn't have children. She's *out.*"

The team agrees, though, to begin an informal campaign for Rebecca Franks, and review her progress in a few weeks. For now the costs will be carried by Harvest Moon. Everyone stands and gathers together their papers and lunch debris, arguing about whose responsibility it is to return the charts to the files. Paula keeps talking to Janet about Rebecca.

"I haven't checked all the possibilities out," she says with her biggest smile, much left unspoken. "She has two doctors who are *supposed* to be taking care of her."

"When I went to nurse's training, I went to a Catholic school and we worked directly with nuns. We did a lot of hands-on stuff. Since I've graduated, Sister Richard is on my shoulder, and the stuff she taught me she's still whispering in my ear. She's still saying, 'Excuse me, but beds need to be kept neat and rooms need to be kept neat, and pills need to be passed in a certain manner. You follow procedure.' So that's how I view professionalism—someone following what they were taught, and not compromising."

The first thing you notice about Janet Krause is her laugh, in all its variety—she has a whinny and a giggle and a chuckle in her repertoire. She laughs at herself and turns a sour, ironic mouth to the foibles of others. But the laugh can disappear very quickly, and in its place is a disapproving frown; she takes slovenliness personally.

Janet is housed in a windowless room once used to store the medication carts. Now carpeted and painted, it is, at six feet square, as carefully planned as an architect's miniature, each chair and plant and picture in place. There is no real alternative, no other office or larger space available. But Janet likes being near the action, as well, being able to see the nurses' station and the hall traffic a few feet away. Her door is often open, brushing against one corner of her desk. The phone on her desk rings frequently; sometimes she will answer it without a word, listen, answer with a single word, and hang up, continuing the interrupted conversation before the connection is broken.

"I took an aptitude test as a child, and my aptitude was to be a general in the army," she says. "And I guess that's what I got to be."

Director of nursing is a self-explanatory title. Janet hires, fires, evaluates, disciplines, and supervises the nurses and the aides. She is solely responsible for schedules—which change constantly, and require endless fine tuning—and is ultimately responsible for the quality of care given by the nursing staff. If a nurse makes an error in treatment, it is Janet's responsibility—to deal with the consequences, and to assure as far as possible that it never happens again. She dresses in street clothes and a lab coat because she doesn't want to be mistaken for the nurses responsible for direct patient care. She sees her role as supervisory, advisory, and almost tangential to bedside care. Now and then a nurse will come to her, stumped, unable to insert a tube or start an I.V., and then Janet will step out onto the floor and help. Occasionally she'll answer a call light as she walks by a room. But her response is likely to be to find the aide or nurse who can fill the request; in the same way, the nurses are more likely to ask each other and the shift supervisors for help with procedures, rather than Janet. She is clearly boss, arbiter of disputes, maker of decisions, the authority.

She has been a nurse for more than twenty years, working in hospitals and in industry, before dropping out of the profession for several years. "I was disillusioned with physicians and the hospital system, the whole thing, and decided I would probably never be a nurse again. I just felt that if you wanted to make changes, you'd probably be butting your head against the wall. Then suddenly I looked around me and realized my kids didn't need me as much as they needed me before, and I decided to look for another job. I still carried with me the bureaucracy of the hospital and how I didn't like it. So I came here. I applied basically because there was an ad in the paper and it was within two miles of my house." She worked as the evening supervisor for two years. "But I spent a lot of time looking around me and saying, 'What happened to professionalism? Why isn't it *here*?' I had had a lot of reservations about longterm care, the lack of professionalism in the staff, the lack of focus on patients' needs, when I first came here. I think it had to do with where I'd come from, hospital-wise."

After the two years on the evening shift, she got restless. "I felt really proud of what I'd accomplished on that shift. Suddenly I found myself wondering what else I could accomplish. I needed to grow, to change." She moved to middle management, and several months ago, after five years at Harvest Moon, became the director of nursing. "Here, you're around the patients, taking care of the patients. This is nursing as it's always been."

She is tall, firm, and unadorned. She dresses plainly in dark dresses and low pumps. Last year, just before her move to the director position, she was selected as the state nursing association's nurse of the year for her involvement in community education.

"I don't know what the future brings," she says. "I know that this facility will get one hundred percent of me all the time

I'm here and probably fifty percent of me when I'm home. I don't even keep track of my hours. I work at home and I don't leave here on time, but I really enjoy it." She has been married for over twenty years and has two teenage girls at home.

It is important to Janet to be fair: "fair and consistent and clear." She gets upset at tardiness, sloppy dress, sarcastic tones of voice. She respects Paula Schulz as a nurse, feels affection toward her, but shakes her head at the many times someone has told her of a particularly Paulaesque comment. In spite of the frequent laughter and obvious satisfaction with herself and her work, Janet has an aloofness in her manner. She is never not the director of nursing, never not aware of the many small and important occurrences around her. When it comes to the residents and their various needs, she is fiercely affectionate, even doting.

This combination of strength and humor serves Janet well in crises, especially the unpredictable crises afforded by the mix of employees and patients under her charge. Last year, Buddy Mullin and Elizabeth Grove, a seventy-six-year-old woman with lung problems who is confined to a wheelchair, became sexual partners.

The Patient's Bill of Rights, a widely disseminated but largely ornamental list of privileges for nursing home patients, mentions conjugal privacy for married couples, but makes no mention of unmarried partners. Buddy and Elizabeth presented a conundrum to the staff. "There were a variety of opinions about whether we should or shouldn't let it happen, *can* we let it happen, and even 'What kind of animals *are* we?' " Janet recalls. "One faction said, '*Look*, a relationship's a relationship, no matter *what* we think. It's not our place to make a decision about that. Our problem is whether or not we can provide them a place where they can meet their needs, physical and emotional.' "

Janet was in firm agreement with that opinion. She helped find a solution: Buddy and Elizabeth were given certain times of the day to use the physical therapy room—with its wide mats set low enough to slide onto from a wheelchair—in privacy. Janet's main problem was helping those employees who felt they couldn't tolerate the relationship to come to terms with it. "Buddy had not been sexually active before, so it was difficult for people in that way. People are very protective of Buddy. They thought this woman was leading him down the garden path." Janet still feels a little impatience at that attitude. She considered renting the movie *Harold and Maude* to show the staff, but the issue cooled before that became necessary. "The other thing, you see, is that they're not married. There was a problem there for the Christians. *I* just think loving is nice—they don't *have* any of that, and how nice for them to be able to get it. How easy for us to forget about it." A few employees have still not forgiven Janet for "encouraging immorality," as she puts it with a smile. "I don't think people totally accepted it," she adds. "But it wasn't our issue at the time. It was theirs. It was for them."

Janet's impatience is sometimes revealed in a distance she places between herself and the nurses and aides she manages. She speaks of herself, at times, in the third person, as "the director of nursing," and of other people by their titles as well: "the nurse practitioner and the director of nursing would do that," she might say. She almost always speaks of her staff with a teacher's detached authority, a constant firm reminder of their existence as a group of workers below her. She says, in praise, "They're doing really well," or "They've made some improvement," and it has a patronizing ring. But there is no real patronizing at work, merely an acceptance of the surface appearance. The aides and nurses don't complain to Janet nearly as often or as vehemently as they complain to each other. They keep their counsel, too, and show only the small disgruntlements of any group of employees. Janet genuinely believes that all is well in her department, because she hasn't been told otherwise.

"At times I think, 'If only I could *show* you this.' But I

know that's not the appropriate way to manage people. I have to let them make their own mistakes and then come for help." She dismisses with an irritated wave the idea that a person could be fired for speaking their mind, for personality conflicts or dissent. She is deeply attached to the idea of professionalism in nursing, standards shared by all who hold the title of nurse, and not by others. Because of this she delineates between the nurses—she calls them "licensed personnel"—and the nurse's aides, who are unlicensed. The lack of formal training, in Janet's mind, means an inability—at least generally—to understand rationale and purpose and long-term goals of nursing care. They persist, she sees, in old habits and time-worn ways, long after the habits are discouraged. When she hears an aide call a patient by an endearment, even by their first name, she stops and openly chastises the employee. Intimacy, even the unparalleled intimacy between strangers that an aide and patient can develop, is no excuse to Janet Krause.

"I hate it," she says. "They should be called 'Mrs. Jones' until they say 'Call me Hazel.' I have really strong feelings that these are *adult human beings*—so what if they have a dementia, they are adults. They are not our peers. They are our elders." She herself slips into the habit of leaning over wheelchairs instead of kneeling at eye level, of patting people on the head or arm and calling them, as is our occasional desire, by names we call children. "I want to *kick* myself! That little pat-on-the-back business." She is laughing now, at her own vehemence, her hectoring tone, but stands firm. "I remember when I was in training we used to say, 'If you think about that being your mother and father, then how would you deal with it?' If that were your parent, how would you want them treated?"

Ten years ago nurses were addressed as "Miss" or "Mrs." or, on occasion, "Nurse"—not only by patients, but by physicians and other nurses. In the casual alliances of the 1980s, almost everyone addresses everyone else by their first name. There are two exceptions common to this: it usually takes a relationship of some involvement to get past the title "Doctor" for the physician. And some nurses still insist, like Janet, on a formal name for the patient. For Janet it goes both ways.

"I wouldn't have any trouble being called 'Mrs. Krause.' But I'm a cap-and-white-uniform person, too. I think a false familiarity isn't always comfortable for people. I had a hard time adjusting to all the first names here. I'd never worked anywhere where people did that before."

CHAPTER FOUR

Little Mercies

"I had a stroke first a ways back and then I fell down and broke my hip." Margaret Bond speaks with a lazy, friendly drawl, the voice of a woman who loves to talk. She talks steadily, quietly, plainly. She has endurance.

"At first, I hated it, to tell the truth. I didn't know anybody. And they took my cigarettes away, which almost killed me!" she laughs. "The first meal we had, they served fish. It was *awful*. Even the cook cried! I called home and said"—she lifts her voice to a whine—"I don't *like* it here!"

Margaret has osteoporosis, which weakens bones and makes them easy to fracture. Under ordinary circumstances the broken hip would have been pinned in place, a straightforward if not simple job, and she would have returned home after several weeks of recovery and therapy. But after a few weeks at Harvest Moon, the pin twisted out of the porous bone, and there is so little solid material left that another may not work. It is November 23 now, and she has already been here for four weeks. She must stay completely off her leg—be, in the local slang, "non-weight-bearing"—while it heals as best it can. "My doctor said, if I could stand it, that twelve or fifteen weeks is what he wanted to start with." She makes a sour face. At the moment she is half "out of whack," one leg worthless and one arm long paralyzed and flaccid from the stroke. Until she fell she had walked with a cane, cooked, kept house for her husband and herself.

Her stay looks to be so long that Nancy Rice encouraged her to go off Medicare—which will pay for only a certain number of days of care a year for any particular problem—until she needs intensive therapy again. Last week she moved from C Wing, the skilled section, to B Wing to wait till she's able to have more therapy. Neither her insurance nor Medicare will pay for intermediate care. The bills are Margaret's sole responsibility.

"That's where we pay the charges," she tells me. "Fifty dollars and fifty cents a day. It isn't doing any good, that's for sure."

Margaret rises as early as the aides are able to help her dress and wash, and she doesn't return to her room until the informal evening curfew at nine P.M. It took a few weeks for Margaret to adjust to the strict smoking policy at Harvest Moon, the product of years of acrimony and failed experiments. Smokers must provide their own cigarettes, kept in a locked cupboard near the nurses' station, and in order to smoke must be at the smokers' table, in the sunny corner of the dining room near the big color television, on the half hour. An aide—a different one each day is entrusted with the key to the cupboard—brings the basket of packs and cartons and distributes one apiece, lights all in a row, and then locks them up again. Curfew follows the last cigarette offered, at eight-thirty in the evening.

"I just sit and yak and read or smoke a cigarette, and then sit and yak some more. All we do is eat, really! I have friends. Lynn, well, she went home, and Elizabeth and Cathy and Robert. Oh, I've made all kinds of friends, and now we've got a new boy at the table. So my kids finally said, 'Aren't you ever coming home, or do you like it that well there?' And I says, 'Well, it ain't like I like it that well, but I don't want to go home until I'm healed, either.'

"My husband, he comes every day. We been married forty-seven years next month. I have three kids, six grandchildren, and a great-grandchild." She shows me a color photograph from the small bag on her lap, of a boy about five years old dressed in a cowboy costume, staring at the camera with intent.

Margaret faces an unexpectedly long time in the company of the same people: she will share the same room with, more than likely, the same two roommates, for many months. Her routine will have little variety beyond what she herself introduces into it, and her personal needs will be looked after, if not always by the same person, by the same rotating group of people with the same information and intent. Those people who care for her will provide the same kind of care to dozens of other people. Such sameness is in the nature of the beast, and it is either tolerated with boredom or enjoyed as a reward. The relationships between nurses, aides, and patients develop a thin edge of exasperation sometimes, shaded with fondness.

Gina Tyrell has very dark skin, accented with heavy purple rouge and a dark wet lipstick. She wears her hair in shiny limp curls that tickle her large tinted glasses with sparkling frames. She is in her early forties and has worked as a nurse's aide at Harvest Moon for seven years. Several years ago she passed a test certifying her as a medication aide, allowed to give medicine—not shots—to patients. Since then she has given out medicine on B and D wings, freeing the practical nurses for more complex duties, and helped answer the phone at the nurses' desk. She plants her stout frame sideways, one girdled hip against the writing surface, and argues with one of her many children on the phone.

"Don't you talk to me like that!" she finally sneers, and slams the receiver down. Gina talks in an exaggerated jive, laughing with a horsey snort. She jokes about everything, claiming always to be on the edge of a breakdown, deflecting serious conversation.

She leans over the desk to speak to an aide, pointing at a

frail old woman in a wheelchair carrying a pair of purple slippers in her lap.

"Will you go talk to that woman 'bout those shoes in her lap?" Gina drawls with scorn. "Woman's been ridin' around with those shoes for three days. Jeeeez."

She shakes her head.

If a nurse or aide learns, in the long months, to love a person, she will either have to say good-bye when the person leaves or be privileged to watch his decline into death. If she comes to dislike—in some cases, dislike passionately—a person, she must still bathe, dress, massage, and feed that person. There is a numbing repetition at work that must not result in numbness; a strict task orientation of items on a list that must not result in task-oriented work. The caregiver—the nurse—must take a total stranger as a wetnurse takes a baby to her breast, without the expectation of gratitude, without the merest certainty that she will be noticed or remembered.

"It don't bother me, the disrespect. If I don't like it, I ain't gonna stay. Some people, you know, they'll ask me, 'How in the world can you stick with a job like *that,* such a dirty job?' I tell them, 'You know, somebody has to do it.' And it has a lot more rewards than people think."

MaryAnn Bigler has worked at Harvest Moon for thirteen years, longer than any other employee. She is thirty-three years old. Her plump face is heavily made up with bright eyeshadow, thick black eyeliner, red lipstick which somehow fails to age her looks past those of a world-worn fifteen-year-old. She wears her fine, curly hair short and pulled back with bright, ribboned barrettes, each bearing a sprig of plastic poinsettia leaves and holly berries. She fills her white stretch pants and the pink smock worn by female aides tightly; the pocket of the smock is decorated with medallions and pins: employee of the year for 1979, the nurse's aide certification pin, small medal clips given in honor of one year's, five years', and ten years' steady employment. In mild defiance of policy, she wears a BORN AGAIN pendant tacked to her lapel. Her eyes are dull and sleepy in her fleshy face and she tells her own kind of war stories.

"I remember this woman, she was paralyzed totally. And she wouldn't let me leave her bedside. I had to sit and hold her hand *every minute* of the day, you know, because she was confused but I was someone she could relate with. Who cared, you know, and she could trust.

"You wouldn't believe the stories I've heard. There was this one woman, Mrs. Jepsen, us girls, we could sit and listen to her for hours on end because of the things she and her husband did at the turn of the century—what this was like and that was like. And this other, Edna Crane, she was a hundred and one years old. There were only two or three of us she let get by calling her by her first name. She *hated* that name. We teased her. That woman was built like a Sherman tank, you know. And it just tickled her to death, we just teased the tar out of her and she loved it! Because, you know, it shows you care. She had a lot to say—back in the turn of the century, the kinds of cars, you know, the changes in the clothing styles, horse and buggy days, you know, are really interesting.

"I think the one I kind of miss the most—what was her name now? She was in Room Forty-three. I can't remember her name, Mary something, it's been a few years. But she worked thirty years in the trainyard, *in the yard* with the men, pushing three-hundred-pound greasecarts around. That woman was strong as an ox and ornery as all get-out.

"You can listen to some of them people and get just as good a history lesson as reading it. It's better than reading—I *hate* reading! I know some people put down the geriatrics because they're senile or this or that, but you stop and think: everything from the past is *still there!* You ask them, everything's intact. Like a human tape recorder. You ask them, and they'll just ramble on. It's amazing."

MaryAnn believes that most of her patients, her "pets," favor her over the other aides. She wears a smile of secrecy, a layer of smug knowledge that she, hidden in anonymity and pink, carries the responsibility of other people's pain and comfort. Most of the aides believe this, and a kind of competition of love is born. After thirteen years of service MaryAnn Bigler makes $5.05 an hour. The competition, however unconscious, is one of the rare rewards.

"So many of the people I take care of, they really like me and they're glad when I'm their aide, and that makes me feel good." John Eldizondo is thirty-five, an ex-medical corpsman in Vietnam and the senior aide on the evening shift. "When I go in Mrs. Mott's room and she finds out I'm gonna be her aide, she grins from ear to ear. And Irma Washington—I'm just about the only person who can make her smile."

"I think about them when I go home." "The smiles, that's your only reward." "I love them." This is the chanted litany in a job of backbreaking labor and repetitive chores. "It's a lousy job. I couldn't last a week. A day," says Bonnie Pereira, a veteran nurse whose responsibilities include making certain the aides perform up to par. The author of a memoir about life in a nursing home called the aides "the real arbiters of our daily destinies." They are responsible for dressing, bathing, "personal care," which includes washing the genitals, brushing teeth, combing hair, and nail care, walking and transferring the patient from bed to chair, transporting patients to activities and therapy, making beds and cleaning up clutter in rooms, toileting and feeding, and taking "vital signs"—temperature, pulse, blood pressure. They also share a number of other responsibilities, such as cleaning up the utility rooms, rinsing and refilling water pitchers, weighing patients, showering patients and helping with therapy baths, and assisting the nurses in dressing changes and other tasks. On B and D wings one aide will be responsible, most days, for ten patients. On C Wing, each also has ten patients, but must contend with fresh wounds, feeding tubes, casts, I.V.s, and the concomitant needs of sicker, less stable patients.

The average length of stay for an aide is between six months and a year. Once the smiles and love are acknowledged, the litany becomes a tired one of quiet, chronic complaint. And all their efforts still leave room for improvement. One patient hisses to me, when I ask her casually how she finds her care: "I haven't been fed, haven't been bathed today. They assume everyone is stone deaf. You're lying there with your eyes closed, trying to rest, and someone comes up and says, 'Hello, dear, how are you?' " She is venomous in her resentment. "It's the most frustrating experience of my life. You can't reach, you can't roll, you can't call. And every time they leave the room, they make sure the table is exactly four inches away from my hand." This woman is confused sometimes; I know she's already been fed. She is hungry and has forgotten the meal. One aide dismisses her with, "She just wants to be pampered." But whether earned or not, such mocking is still painful.

"I've tried many times to understand why the aides are so short-term. Why is their dedication and devotion to the patients so up and down?" wonders Janet Krause, who worked briefly as an aide while in nursing school. She is unsure how to voice the conviction, though it troubles her, but she suspects the aides are often aides because it is a job within their socioeconomic class, a reflection of the low skills, poor education, and lack of options of people doomed to little more than poverty. "It's an entry-level position. They know that salaries are low, that you can't support yourself or your family on the salary."

Barb Coulter, the part-time speech therapist, watches the aides work with a kind of morbid fascination. "People who don't know what else to do or can't do anything else, take jobs that aren't very appealing to other people. I'm not sure many of the nurse's aides enjoy their jobs over the years. There is really no way to make that job nice, doing not-nice things."

Janet Krause says she "paid her dues" as an aide long ago.

Paula Schulz, remembering her first job, alone in the three-story building in Minnesota, has little patience with the griping. As Janet puts it, it is an "entry-level" position. Who would stay in such a job—stay for years, moving from nursing home to nursing home as many do—if not someone with no other choices?

"If every RN including Janet would just stoop down to my level," says John Eldizondo, one of the most vocally unhappy aides, "and just be an aide, no strings attached, for eight hours every six months, it would do them a world of good."

"When I was younger I wanted to be a nurse. That was four years ago. But just being an aide and being around the nurses—they have too much work to do, and too little time. And I think the aides have it worse than the nurses. You don't have any time to socialize with the patients. You don't have any time for one-to-one contact. You just whip in and whip out. They don't get any companionship, really." Mickey Bestler is twenty-four now. She goes to school two days a week to become a legal secretary, and works three days a week at Harvest Moon, where she has been employed off and on for four years. She is thin, brash, and likes to lean lazily against a wall, chewing on the toothpick eternally between her large front teeth. She calls herself "a party animal," then giggles about cooking dinner for her boyfriend. She wears thick makeup, shrouds her eyes in eyeliner and mascara. She is actually fast and efficient at her work, and seems to enjoy the irritated looks Janet and the other nurses throw at her when they find her loitering. Mickey is unrepentant, obdurate, secure in her years of experience and the columns of help-wanted ads begging for nurse's aides elsewhere. She is amused by the management's continuing efforts to fuel loyalty to Harvest Moon itself.

"The management is loyal because they're the ones making all the money. I'd be loyal, too, if I was making twelve bucks an hour. There *is* a difference," she declares, pointing with her toothpick. Mickey makes $4.40 an hour on the day shift, and is often assigned, by virtue of her skills, to the back section of C Wing, the heaviest care assignment in the building.

"There's a lot of people who work here as aides that I would not even *consider* an interview with. They're just hiring people who aren't going to make waves, people who don't care, who mask their work. On the surface they're great, but if you were to follow them around behind the curtains, you would know *different*.

"The structure to me seems to be that they want to deal with the problems that arise so that they always get changed around to be something they're not," Mickey adds, confident in her meaning. "If it's something that *we* feel is really important, they act like we're making something big out of nothing, and they're going to handle it and we're never going to hear anything about it."

Odd, that caring for our fellows' most intimate needs is considered unskilled labor. The low compensation reflects the hard-won view of the professionals that work of the mind, performed behind a desk, is more difficult than work performed by hands and muscles. The other, less tangible requirements, the Horatio Alger, seat-of-the-pants education, is rarely articulated. The first lessons of an aide are ones of shocking intimacy. The duties are private, cold splashes not of sameness, but of difference: differences of gender, age, health, and physical decay. "When I was first an aide, it was like, 'Oh, God, this is really personal!' " says Mickey. "Now I think that everybody in high school should do this kind of work for a month. I think that they'd look at elderly people in a different way, that they would know more about themselves and how life really goes."

There is truth in the assumption that people work as nurse's aides because they haven't any choice. It is a relatively easy job to get; most, but not all, employers require certification, which can be obtained in about six weeks at a cost of about $100. Though the pay is low—usually little over minimum wage—it is a highly secure position. Janet hires and fires two, three, sometimes four aides a month. But the ones fired—always, says Janet, for poor performance and nothing else—are likely to have new aide jobs within a week, without references. The rapid turnover reflects the dissatisfaction and restlessness of the employees, who can pick and choose from dozens of help-wanted ads every day. It is better work, perhaps, than processing thousands of long-distance calls, working a cannery line, or sitting in front of a display terminal for hours. I suspect a lot of cannery workers would despise nurse's aide work. It is in the eye of the beholder, when there *are* choices. But because people enter with few qualifications and often no experience in other work, there is almost no hope of promotion. Aides don't supervise, teach, schedule, budget, order supplies, or even organize paperwork. The only skills you will learn as a nurse's aide are those of an aide.

Many nurses, including myself, started as aides. We had options, the niceties of college tuition and high school educations. We became nurses for one of two curiously parallel reasons: either because we enjoyed the work and wanted to know more, to be able to do more, or we couldn't stand the work and needed another skill. One of the professors in my nursing school, a vocal proponent of "professionalizing" nursing, said she didn't trust nurses who had started as aides. She considered it a disadvantage, afraid that we would misunderstand the nature of nursing, think it was mostly physical tasks at the bedside instead of the application of theory.

A very few people climb the ladder. The supply coordinator at Harvest Moon started as an aide. A few assistant cooks have started as kitchen aides, and the admissions coordinator started as a clerk. Promotion creates a curious boundary: the few so honored quickly reach a point where they stop complaining about the working conditions and start explaining them. It is moot to the aides who must punch in and out for every scheduled fifteen-minute break, who take half-hour lunches when told it is time, now, to go, who come to work at six forty-five in the morning and perform at the assignment handed them.

Each month at the general staff meeting where paychecks are distributed, employees are asked to vote for an employee of the month. Once a year one of these twelve is chosen as employee of the year, and given a pin and a shake of the hand. The honorees are photographed for the bulletin board in the main hall. The flash batteries in the old Polaroid are weak. Caught at the end of a shift, the employees look sallow and tired in the yellow light it casts. Now, in November, a circle of dark-rimmed eyes above white uniforms, the brown smocks of housekeeping and the blue tops of the kitchen workers, covers the board. Roger Scarpelli thinks it's "nice" to do such things, but scorns the need for it: "I feel that when you take a job on, you take the responsibility on. You're gonna do the job and for that you're compensated. That's a bargain you make. The other odds and ends—I have a difficult time with it. People look for rewards. For trinkets."

Of such is the disparity between labor and management made. Behind a desk, the management can remember with fondness the dues paid in the past. They feel secure in their imagination of the laborer's life, certain they understand with the wisdom of years. So Janet Krause can see the fast turnover, see unhappy faces, arguments over the schedule, and wonder why their "devotion and dedication to the patients" changes.

The day-shift nursing supervisor post is a position of critical importance at Harvest Moon. The person in the position coordinates the care of all the patients, communicates with physicians and families, does admissions and discharge paperwork, teaching, scheduling, and supervision.

The longtime supervisor quit last month, and Janet quickly hired a replacement. But the new nurse lasted only a few weeks in the position before being transferred, rather ignobly, to the night shift.

"You get one or two nurses like her and you ruin your relationship with the docs," Paula tells me, out of Janet's hearing. "She was calling them two or three times a day for nothing at all. I tell you, the lights are on and nobody's home."

"I have a real problem with Paula's way of talking," Janet responds later, when I give her an edited version of Paula's remarks. "It's a real problem here, that she is *not* a nursing administrator. Her job is managing patient care, not running the nurses." Janet is trying to be careful, to speak with tact. But she is upset; she sees Paula's lack of discretion as almost a personal affront. "She's very good with patients. Exceptionally good. But there is a lot of"—Janet pauses to consider the right word—"*conversation* right now about role definition."

Judy Currie graduated from nursing school six months ago and came to work as a floor nurse on C Wing. Janet is trying to convince her to take the supervisory position, which rotates between all the RNs until someone is hired. Bonnie Pereira, the senior nurse on day shift after four years, has no desire for the promotion. "People throw information at you, and you call a doc and they take a message and never call back," she says in amused exasperation. "I like to have my own place, my own little area. I *choose* to stay there."

Judy feels inadequate to the job. She is a tall, slender, thirty-five-year-old woman, a homemaker and the mother of two children until a divorce several years ago landed her unexpectedly in the job market. She became a nurse's aide, saw it had no future, and went to nursing school.

"I really had a reality shock," she says of the several months she has worked at Harvest Moon. She is carefully groomed, wearing a frilled pillbox nurse's cap on her neat, short hair. She holds herself straight, a picture of conscientiousness and responsibility. "I couldn't believe how much I was being asked to do, how many people I was being asked to care for. I really had a crisis after a time. Everyone else seemed to be doing okay, getting everything done. I wondered what was wrong with me, that it seemed so overwhelming."

Gradually, Judy learned to organize her work. She saw that no one really finished all their chores, that everyone was overwhelmed at times. She is becoming not only more efficient, but more confident, and agreed to try supervising on occasion. If she thinks she can handle it, after a month, she'll take the job.

Gerry Kennett is dying of ovarian cancer. She is fifty-four years old; for many years she and her husband ran a store together. Now he is dead. "I'm an authority," she says, lips cracked and dry, her voice no louder than her whispery breath. "I had a sister in a nursing home. I had a mother in a nursing home. I had a husband in a nursing home. I know all about them."

She is fed by a tube threaded through her nose, down her throat into her stomach. Every few hours a nurse pours a few cups of formula into the plastic bag hung on a pole beside her bed; the formula slowly drips down the tube. Many times Paula and the floor nurses have taken out her tube and tried to help Gerry Kennett eat; she invariably vomits. Several times she has asked that the tube be removed, expressing the desire to die, then relents, afraid that without it she *would* die. The team is discouraged; she is months from death, but until the tube comes out she can't go home. Of the line that leashes her to Harvest Moon, she says only, "You get used to hanging if you hang long enough."

This trace of bitter humor is the only sparkle Gerry shows. She spends her days sleeping, watching game shows on television, occasionally talking with the one friend who visits her. She usually must lie flat on her back to control the nausea.

"It is absolutely top of the mark as far as boredom is concerned. Some people are perfectly wonderful, others brutal. Nothing for me to do. So much for them to do and so many people," she says, with a tiny crooked smile, her head capped with very short, iron-gray hair. "You ring the bell and nobody comes."

Her bed is beside the window that fills the whole southern wall, opening to the brick courtyard, still, after years, unfinished. In the courtyard is a metal table with several metal chairs and a sun umbrella hanging on its pole. It sits beside a barbecue pit. The bricks end halfway to the high cyclone fence at the back of the property, empty except for two unpruned pear trees. In the winter rain it is a scene of emptiness, of lawn furniture forgotten long after the family has retreated to the living room. In the summer, unimaginably distant, the curtains must be drawn to keep out the heat.

Here all the "conversation" between managers, all the petty and serious arguments and theories, fall short. This is the bed, the nest, the stopping place. It has its own vocabulary, its own tang in the air, its own priorities. The priorities are often so different, so unusual to the healthy who walk nearby, that they are forgotten—with a casual, unintended neglect, a simple pre-occupation with other matters, with things that need doing.

An old, silent woman occupies the other bed in the room, nearer the door. When I arrive today to see Gerry, late in the morning, the curtain is drawn around that bed and I step by. But as I pass the end I see the curtain isn't drawn all the way. The woman sits on the side of her bed, naked. She is thin; her deserted breasts hang limply to her navel. She mutely meets my gaze. The aide standing beside her, rolling up the sleeves of a housedress before pulling it over the woman's head, looks at me with an almost identical blankness. I pass the tableau to Gerry's bed, Gerry's small habitat, and it is as though the scene had never occurred. It is timeless, endless, meaningless.

Gerry talks about her son—"a wonderful guy but completely immature"—and how she worries what will happen to him when she dies. Her cancer was a shock; she had never been sick. She knows she has "no future," and the mocking venom with which she sometimes attacks the nurses only lasts a while before it recedes into the gray.

"You feel like a beetle on its back." She twists a little in bed, tugging at the feeding tube. "A beetle on its back."

CHAPTER FIVE

The Staff of Life

A horrible gurgling shriek flies down the hallway, landing at the nurses' desk as though dropped from a height. Nancy Rice looks at Judy Currie, sitting beside her. "Who was that?" she asks, tired, only mildly concerned. "It's been so long since we've had a screamer."

Gertrude Werner is sitting beside the desk in a wheelchair. She has been using it more often lately. "Honey, what's the matter?" she asks, sniffing the air.

Judy leans toward her. "She's having some therapy and she doesn't like it." Another scream pushes its way through the hall.

"Is that all?" Gertrude is full of disdain. "Honey, you have to stop crying." She rolls herself toward the sound rapidly, raising her voice. "Now you have to be quiet!" she adds to the din, determined to be heard. "You sound like you got your neck broken!"

Paula's "special case," Rebecca Franks, died this morning, of a sudden pneumonia which filled her lungs like a tide. "She was old," Paula says matter-of-factly, not without sadness. "I don't think we failed her. We would have failed her if we hadn't tried—if we'd given her up like they told us to."

By the dining room door Max Kleiner is pushing Phoebe White in her wheelchair, back and forth in a semicircle beside him. "Bay-bay-bay," he hums, rolling her to and fro in a slight curve. "Bay-bay-bay," a lullaby which she accepts in silence as she slides along.

The small activity room is attached to the end of C Wing. It looks out on the bricked patio. Charlene Parrott has her occupational therapy equipment here, Margery Todd her activities desk. There is a shelf of big-print books and *Reader's Digests*, a television, a refrigerator where families and friends keep special treats for patients. In a large wire cage lives a big white rabbit named Houdini.

Today the doors are closed, a curtain partly drawn. Once a month this room is given over to Mass. A small horseshoe of people faces a Formica table topped with a flickering candle and a silver chalice. Behind the table sits a large, stolid man, bald, silent, his eyes closed behind thick glasses. He is robed in the dress of a priest. The whole room is silent, in a curious suspension, and then the priest's lips begin to move and he starts the blessing. He is calling down a miracle, and a solemn, joyous tension fills the room, emptied of its daily, trudging routine. For a short while the huge question of life and death and afterlife that shadows that routine is brought to the surface. In the big cluttered room it is acknowledged, even embraced, then laid to rest in tacit silence for a while more.

Howie Kramer is a Catholic, but he rarely goes to Mass. Of late he rarely goes anywhere at all.

His fat, baby-round face matches the childish whine with which he speaks. Howie Kramer has a very odd voice: it is tight, as though he talked through a strained, thick throat, but blurred and mushy, too, with halved words and sliced-off consonants. He speaks slowly, with the stupid languor of one almost asleep.

He has been lying on his back for eighteen years. He has multiple sclerosis, a degeneration of the nervous system that shaves the insulation off the neural wires, until the body becomes a weird panorama of sparking circuits. It paralyzes, tightens, spasms, and hurts. This accounts for the dull, tight quality of his voice, and, in part, for the rambling, trivial discourses he treats any and all visitors to, full of irrelevancies and unexpected changes of topic. Howie tends to focus on one thing—always a personal problem—and return to it again and again in the course of a conversation. Howie's consciousness is so fragmented now that even his free association is jerky and frayed.

"I'm all alone. Nobody cares about me." Howie says this often. Sometimes it's his daughter who doesn't care about him; sometimes it's Paula or Nancy. He envisions a large conspiracy of the uncaring to account for his miseries, for the constant frustrations that populate his life.

"Stuck between the dark blue sea and the devil, I guess," he tells me. "That's an old phrase, how old do you think *I* am?" I've known him for three years, but he doesn't always remember this. "I'm forty-eight years old. I feel old. I feel old, old, old."

His limbs and spine are twisted into a shape vividly known as the "wind-blown posture." Both knees are drawn up and thrown far to one side as though in a sudden gale; one elbow is also doubled up. His tendons have contracted in spasms for so many years that they have actually shortened, drawn up as though the seamstress had taken up the hem. Tendons can be cut in surgery, to ease such contractions, but Howie's veins and arteries have shortened, too. Eighteen years is a long time.

He worked as a computer programmer for IBM, entering programs into the huge, expensive, finicky machines of the past era. He forgets, now, what and how he did that. I tell him about personal computers, desk-top keyboards, and he is surprised—surprised in the flat, unsurprised way he feels everything but pain.

"I was married for seven and a half years. I know it's not very long. My wife is married for the third time now. I was only twenty-two when I got married. Too damned young. And she was even younger, nineteen. But it was okay, or so I thought. I don't remember. It's been so long since I seen her. This disease," he finishes, "just gets worse and worse." His conversation travels small peaks and valleys of interest and despair. Every few minutes it doubles back to his repeated and echoing days. "I'll *never* get any sleep. I've started haw-loo-sinn-ating. Darn right. And my doctor won't do anything about it, neither."

Howie has a daughter who is twenty-one years old now. She lives an hour's drive away, but has visited him only once, briefly, in eight years. He has a son, too. "He never did a single thing I told him to do," mourns Howie. "But I loved him anyway." He has not seen his son in over five years, does not know his whereabouts. His mother is his only other relative, an invalid who calls Howie every day without fail—till recently. She is in the hospital and her calls have been irregular. "She has art-a-ritis so bad. She humps over. She can't call because she probably doesn't have a phone. I can't call her 'cause I don't know where she is. They won't even tell me."

I suggest to Howie that he talk with Nancy Rice about his mother, and see if she could help him get in touch. "She won't help," he chants. "She's against me, too."

Howie has, for several years, refused the physical therapy exercises which would have kept him in a more normal posture, which would, even now, ease the stiffness and pain. The exercises hurt, he says. He refuses even the hot packs to his joints which ease the constant aching that is part disease and part immobility. He looks, huddled up in bed under a single neatly tucked-in sheet, as wide as he is long. He refuses baths and shampoos, clean sheets, toothbrushing. Howie's skin glistens with sweat and oil, his hair is stringy. He shares the room with Buddy Mullin, the young man with brain damage. The door to the hall is covered with a Pat Benatar poster, the bathroom door decorated with a Garfield cartoon poster. Buddy's massing of stereo equipment, garnered over the years as gifts, lines the far walls. But the room smells sour and unsavory, the smell of human illness and failure. In the last year Howie has gained over fifty pounds, and is far too heavy and ungainly to be lifted now. He can only be lifted with a Hoyer lift, a kind of hydraulic jack with a linen basket specifically designed for people like Howie. He dislikes the Hoyer and often refuses it, claiming that it hurts, that he is afraid he will fall.

Howie Kramer wasn't always as he is now. For years he kept to himself in a quiet, meditative way, calm and accepting of his care, gently refusing offers of distraction or company. For years Margery Todd, the activity director, brought him hamburgers and french fries and milkshakes several times a week, knowing it was bad for his weight, but unable to resist his childish pleading. Now his weight is a serious problem, and hamburgers are no longer on the menu. He often refuses Margery's visits, or the little card games she offers to play with him. Occasionally he will attend a musical program or church, but he grows more capricious almost daily.

"He is *extremely* difficult," Janet Krause admits. "And I think we all understand why. We tried spending a lot of time with him and what we got was Howie wanting someone with him all the time. We take turns dealing with it."

"Here's this guy," says Paula, who remembers Howie's happier days, "who's been cheery and smiling for all these people for years and has been left to lie there without much attention, and then he gets sick and feels cranky and all of a sudden people are going in there twelve times a day. He's not going to give up that behavior. Why *should* he give up that behavior? It works. Clinically, he's stable. It doesn't have anything to do with his disease. It has to do with lying on your back for eighteen years."

But Paula gets annoyed with him, too, and answers him abruptly or not at all when he makes bizarre demands. Willie, the dishwasher famous for his ability to wheedle smiles out of difficult patients, rolls his eyes when it comes to Howie. "Heavens, don't give me him," he says. "He's just a big baby. That's what I tell him, 'You're a big baby.' I mean, come *on*—he wants to take baths in *mineral water?* I said, 'Come *on!*' "

Mineral water baths are only one of the demands he has made, and Willie neatly summarizes the feelings of many. Some of the staff are ready to give up on Howie Kramer, and they can't. He's here, he needs help, his demands are both petulant and pathetic. He is a perpetually ill, manipulative child. He is afraid. He has looked at the ceiling and a small, dusty, yellow curtain for most of the last eighteen years. In a way Howie Kramer is beyond the pale—he has failed to meet the social contract, he *can't* meet the social contract any more. It has been so long since he has been able to interact in a remotely equal fashion with people, so long since he has been distracted from the eccentric irritations of his body for more than a moment, that he has forgotten how. All he has to talk about any more is his own misery.

"I can't do anything, I get so bored," he tells me, as I settle on the foot of his bed. Howie stirs in me a measure of tenderness, atop an interest of a more clinical kind. But he oppresses me, his smells and his chants of self and loneliness, even as I feel guilty for my response. As we talk an aide brings the lunch tray, and I offer to feed Howie, allowing the aide to leave with obvious relief.

"I won't eat egg salad. I won't eat the vegetables either," he says, glancing at the tray. "I won't eat the pears, because I don't like them, either. I know I'm too damned fussy. But they won't give me anything I like." This week Howie asked for egg salad, for every meal. He has asked specifically for pears.

"I'll never accept this. I'm better off dying. Dying may not be so bad." He stares at the lunch tray and summons a transparent bravado, but he can't hold on to it, it slips away like everything else. "Of course, I worry about it. But then again, I don't." He looks at me, a real question in his face this time. "If I go fast, it won't hurt, will it?" I shake my head. "Am I shouting?" he asks, in the same querulous, worried voice.

Barbie Moscowitz gave notice a few weeks ago; Thanksgiving is her last day at Harvest Moon, after three steady years. Unlike a lot of dieticians working in health care, Barbie has experience as a chef's assistant in a prestigious restaurant. She also has a degree in business administration alongside her degree in food service. She has grown bored with the problems of management, the bickering of personnel conflicts, and the niggardly budgeting of the kitchen. When she unexpectedly received an offer in food sales at a starting salary higher than what she earns now, she had no regrets about accepting it.

"About two months ago I was swearing up and down geriatrics was my area," she says, leaning back in her office chair in the midst of confusion. Files, papers, and cans of food are strewn on nearly every surface. A tin labeled DEHYDRATED WATER sits atop the file cabinet. "But none of them are happy. They complain about the food. They're really hard to please. You figure you please them if you don't get a lot of complaints. It's not because the cooks are getting patted on the back or anything, it's just because you're not hearing any complaints."

The kitchen is a high-ceilinged place, hot and cold by turns as you pass steam tables, walk-in coolers, and large, square, shiny machines of unknown function, unknown control, that fuss and shake without warning. Everything is outsized: the blender holds several quarts, the soup kettles gallons. The shelves are lined with dusty gallon jars of thyme leaves, parsley flakes, black pepper. On one is a large plastic squeeze bottle of "dark egg yolk liquid food color," used to make macaroni and cheese yellow. Noises are soft, harsh, in turns—the whoosh of steam escaping, the clatter of dishes. Fifty-gallon garbage cans are scattered in the corners.

"At six o'clock in the morning the aides start bringing us coffee and some kinda roll and juice," says Margaret Bond with satisfaction, listing the events of the day. The routine is demarcated by food. "Then between nine and nine thirty, they serve breakfast, twelve or twelve thirty we have lunch, then five or six we have dinner, and then we go back to our rooms at night, except I don't go back until after the eight thirty cigarette, and get in bed, then there's another snack sitting there waiting for us! No wonder I've gained nine pounds."

All this bounty is declared necessary by the state, which dictates that "nourishment" be offered to patients five times every day. Many of the lucky fail to appreciate the gesture; a distressingly large portion of the "continental snack"—a sweet roll or piece of toast and coffee or juice—is thrown away untouched day after day. It is served long before many people are awake, and cold by the time they are ready to eat—or someone is ready to feed them. But the state has spoken, and the waste is a necessary loss. A row of microwaves might solve the problem of temperature, but one is all Harvest Moon can afford, and it is often broken. Who would stand and wait? There's work to be done.

The kitchen is Doris Garland's domain. She is day cook. Today's menu is chicken apricot, rice pilaf, zucchini, and angel food cake, chosen from an endlessly rotating menu calendar by Barbie Moscowitz, the dietician.

"Now I come in, in the morning, and start my celery and potatoes for the soup for lunch, and that's cooking while I make the sandwiches. Then I make the soup while the chicken's starting to thaw for supper. Then of course it's time for lunch." Doris works while she talks, or talks while she works; it is hard sometimes to separate the two. She is mixing a sweet sauce for the chicken breasts: two cans of apricot nectar, two cups of light corn syrup, a dollop of corn starch, and a sprinkle of ginger. "After lunch I make this sauce for the chicken, like I'm doing now, and let it sit, and mix up the rice pilaf which has to cook for fifty-five minutes, and while that's in I can cook two pork roasts for tomorrow. Now, normally, I'd do Thursday's dinner tomorrow but Thursday's a holiday, so I'll do the dressing and spice the turkeys today."

On Thanksgiving, employees are given a free meal, and family members are invited to join their relatives for a dinner laid out on tables covered with linen tablecloths. It is not, of course, real linen: linen is too expensive, too difficult to clean. But it is linen in intent.

"Now I have to get the chicken out and into the warmer while Tasha cuts the cake and sets up," Doris adds as she shifts a tray. Tasha is a blushing, brown-skinned girl half-hidden by the ovens. She lays out six plates at a time in front of her, slices a piece of angel food cake onto each plate, garnishes it with coconut, and swiftly wraps it in plastic. At the mention of her name she glances up, smiles, and hurriedly returns to work.

Doris is short and wears thick glasses. She was named employee of the year two years ago and tried to refuse it, claiming she didn't deserve the honor. ("I didn't handle it very well," she admits now.) As the afternoon passes, her glasses steam over and she repeatedly wipes them clean; she is never still, moving between pans and machines like a bee at flowers. She rips open two six-pound packages of frozen zucchini slices and drops them, plop, into trays, then slides the trays into a steamer.

Judy Currie brings the diet order on a patient just admitted. Each patient's diet must be ordered by his or her physician; food supplements, vitamins, even beer and wine must be ordered before they are allowed. There are many and varied diets, which in practice translate to the same foods in different forms, made of slightly different things: soft, made of easily chewed foods; puree, in which ordinary foods are put through a blender (I have seen, in other nursing homes, entire tuna-fish and peanut-butter sandwiches blended, to be spooned out as a kind of pudding); two-gram-sodium diets, with restricted salt; diabetic diets, with restricted carbohydrates and proteins—usually restricted in calories as well—and liquid diets, thin or thick, with jello, sodas, broths, and milks depending on the strictness.

Tasha brings three towering, wheeled carts to the front of the steam tables where Doris works. She opens the doors, revealing the shelves inside, and begins to lay out trays, plates, silverware, napkins and glasses. While Doris dishes up the food for each patient, following a little diet card that also lists preferences (no eggs, coffee with each meal), Tasha fills the beverage request and packs the cart. She is only seventeen, and utterly silent, a small embarrassed smile on her face, shiny in the heat.

"I didn't used to have any help in here till four thirty but the patients are getting so complicated now I just couldn't do it. It takes a lot of concentration all the time," says Doris, still mixing foods. Another dark young woman with an Asian face is pureeing peaches in the giant blender.

"And of course I have to know the people who don't like chicken—I have Swiss steak for them." She drops a dozen frozen patties, gravy attached to each in a solid plate, onto a tray, then slides it into the steamer. In her last act of preparation she grinds several cups of chicken cubes and a cup of apricot sauce together, to replace the chicken for the puree diets. Buddy Mullin, whose preferences are well known, has a pan for himself of beef ravioli.

"Ruby can't chew so well any more. I think she just gets tired, actually," Doris says of a longtime resident. "She prefers ground meat. And her stomach can't handle spicy foods any more." Doris's glasses are coated with steam. She pauses to wipe them clean.

It is hours more before she leaves; Doris must make certain the pots are washed, the leftovers put away. She must glance at the next day's menu, check for its ingredients, be certain there are no surprises waiting in the morning. Her husband is a diabetic, a "brittle" one whose condition is erratic and constantly changing. When she leaves Harvest Moon, Doris heads home to cook his supper, sort out the food in her own kitchen, and plan his snacks, his meals, for tomorrow.

66

CHAPTER SIX

"With my angels Sugar Kitten by my side"

For three days the wind has been blowing without relief. In the last days of November the steady rain turned to snow, but last night the snow turned into tiny cubes of ice, each a pristine crystal unconnected to its fellows. The wind blew the sparkling ice sideways along the street, piling it up against curbs and porches in shining, mirrored drifts that tinkle a little as they shift. It is thoroughly December, indisputably winter. By noon the cars in the open, unprotected parking lot at Harvest Moon are coated with a rippled layer of rock-hard frosting. The ice thickens steadily; nothing changes in the sky.

In care conference Nancy Rice, the social worker, sits down resignedly.

"I have a lot of hopeless cases here," she says to the gathering group. "Can I just write 'hopeless case, no future planning'? Then we can all go home."

Judy Currie smiles, a little shy still in her new role as the nursing supervisor. "I hope it snows twenty-four inches as soon as I get home. I'm expendable—no one's going to be discharged in twenty-four inches of snow."

Paula Schulz eyes her seriously over her glasses. "But *I'm* going to be here to discontinue their Medicare coverage."

"I wonder when it's going to break through," says Nancy, gazing at the noontime dusk.

"Next spring," replies Paula.

It is harder for the patients to be philosophical about the weather. In the unbroken tedium of the routine, visitors, mail, activities hold sway. When the winter harumphs and rolls over, settling across town like a giant, lazy dog, then visitors don't arrive. The mail is delayed, activities are canceled—and the already strained staff ends up working short.

In the humdrum of the repeated days, where even television is uncertain—for patients must provide their own televisions, must convince relatives or friends somehow to buy or loan a television for the bedside table, for that hour of "Wheel of Fortune" that sparks each day—therapy schedules are an oasis of interest and variety. Therapy provides not only work, but a goal, a purpose to the days. "Total rehabilitation" is more than the hope of stronger legs or more flexible fingers. It is a schedule, a routine, an expectation—a responsibility. It is a reason to wake up, to wash one's face, climb out of bed, and wheel down the hall.

In the physical therapy room across the intersection from the nurses' desk, Tillie Mott is walking—in a fashion. Almost two months ago Mrs. Mott had a stroke, leaving her paralyzed on the right side. She can now walk eight steps, balanced between two bars, twice a day. A therapy aide stands near her, urging her toward the full-length mirror at the end of Tillie's path, the mirror that is supposed to guide her use of the paralyzed leg. She must drag the leg forward and place it straight before her with every step. They are long, painful ones, eight altogether, until Tillie Mott backs again into the wheelchair with gratitude.

Like many stroke victims, Mrs. Mott is confused and has trouble speaking. Her voice is muffled and round, the consonants blurring into long vowels, deep and slurred. The aide asks her how she feels. Mrs. Mott stares at her hands.

"I'm naked and I'm cold," she answers.

Eight hours a day, five days a week, and half of Saturday, the four therapy assistants—three of whom are licensed physical therapy assistants who have completed two years of college in the field—follow the same schedule. Each has her own list of patients and each patient has a list of exercises and skills to practice determined by Martin King, the physical therapist. Therapy sessions are the most important part of the day for many of the patients on C Wing—victims of strokes, people recovering from total hip replacements or hip fractures. One person may be assigned to walk down the hall with a walker, twice a day, and practice moving from a bed to a chair for twenty minutes. Another may work on toe stretches and ankle turns to improve strength and flexibility. These simple goals are enormous and complex, and sometimes hover just beyond reach with infuriating seduction.

Many people, eager for progress and the promised return home, will hurry through their morning meal in order to be waiting in the therapy room when their turn comes. Others must be sought. Still others are bedridden, like Howie Kramer with his multiple sclerosis. The aides go to them, and stretch and massage the joints and forgotten limbs to ease their stiffening and liven the skin and muscle. When it is young Buddy Mullin's turn, twice a day, he rises suddenly to his height of six and a half feet, hands strapped to the handles of a walker, and stiffly, rapidly strides the length of the longest hallway, twice a day, every day. Every single day. Between these sessions the aides make notes on each person's progress, compare techniques, chat.

"No greater reward can ever be given than man's service and humanity to man. To this Physical Therapy department this reward should be first-rate evidence for rendering such service." So begins a typed letter, framed and hung with care at eye level by the door. It was written last year by an elderly man named Phillips, a healthy and exuberant man who had been run over by a car and been sent to Harvest Moon for the resulting months of recovery. "I know everyone by name," he wrote.

"Do you believe I ever called one by name? No, it was Sugar, Sugar Pudding, Baby, Honey Kitten. Always a name of a child's delight. The closest thing to heaven on earth is a child. Their glowing response to every patient was that of a child."

Phillips was badly injured by the car, and his hips suffered the most. Both were pinned in intricate surgeries, and he worked hours every day, in considerable pain, to strengthen them. Twice a pin slipped out of place, and he had to return to surgery. On his last day in Harvest Moon, against the orders of his doctor and the advice of the physical therapist, he walked a few steps from his wheelchair to a friend's car. The new pin snapped out of the bone like a door kicked off its hinges. After that Phillips was in the hospital for weeks.

"My dear and one of my best friends, Brian, I hate to say this," Phillips continued in his letter, addressing the former physical therapist. "He is much too handsome and a fine gentleman to be in his predicament. He is a poor Yankee fan, poor fellow. Now if he would just come over to the Dodgers he would have half the world in his hand."

I took my young son to see Phillips in the hospital, bearing a bowl of homemade soup and a bag of candy for his well-known sweet tooth. He was propped up against a mound of pillows, his skin a black sheen, his teeth bared with pleasure at the sight of visitors. He ignored the treats in favor of a little boy he'd never met before, his big hands reaching out in welcome. "Ah, hello!" he called. Phillips spent a long while in that bed, and the hospital didn't send him back to Harvest Moon. Perhaps they blamed the home for Phillips's troubles. At any rate, they kept him there until he was able to go home, hobbled for life with a bad limp but undeterred. Sometime later he wrote the letter.

"P.S. I almost forgot," he finished. "I don't feel no ways tired, I have come too far from where I started from. Nobody told me that the road would be easy. With my angels Sugar Kitten by my side I know God had not brought me this far to leave me."

Martin King, the physical therapist, is the essential mild-mannered man: short and slim, his hair thinning on top, with a neat mustache and glasses. He is never seen without a tie, never ruffled, and he never raises his voice. His desk is free of clutter, the walls near his workspace carefully decorated with posters of a man in various stages of undress: first the man's muscles, then his nerves and blood vessels are seen; and at last he is exposed in all his skeletal glory.

It is Martin's job to run the entire department, and he is the only physical therapist on duty. He does all the assessments, writes plans and exercise programs, evaluates each person's progress regularly, schedules and supervises the aides and reads their notes, attends conferences and consultations, teaches, and makes discharge plans. He keeps track of the number of treatments he and his staff perform: in November they administered over seven hundred sessions of physical therapy. He is obviously burdened by the load, but is too polite to say so in such a bald way. "There's a lot, sure," he says. "I guess maybe there's more to do than I realized."

Half an hour of physical therapy costs $20; an evaluation is $60. Many stroke victims are old enough to be covered by Medicare, but not all. Harvest Moon is obliged by law to charge private-pay patients the same charge billed to Medicare. But, as in many non-profit homes, sympathy can win over propriety. People often lose their Medicare coverage, which is limited to a certain period of time in certain circumstances, before they are beyond help. Most stroke patients, in fact, can continue to benefit from regular therapy for the rest of their lives, and it can't always be provided by a family member. "The facility gives away a lot of treatments, a lot of evaluations. I let the administration know how many I'm giving away just to keep tabs, and they're very supportive. It's not going to make or break us, because we're always getting more Medicare rehab patients whom we can charge the full rate."

The range of possible results from therapy is broad and often unpredictable; but the results are rarely, if ever, negative.

The results, too, are directly tied to the intensity and frequency of the therapy sessions: two sessions a day of twenty minutes each are far more beneficial than a session of an hour twice a week. Most people who receive efficient, professional therapy benefit notably. "Success is really individual," says Martin King. "For some people it might be to transfer independently. For another it might be to walk with a cane. And for another it might be buttoning a shirt." Martin and his assistants learned long ago not to be fooled by outward appearances, never to imagine that age or medical diagnosis can predict the final result. Each day brings surprises.

Custer Holland is one of the surprises. At eighty-seven, with obstructive lung disease, poor circulation, painful legs, congestive heart failure, and high blood pressure, he is a victim of his own longevity and the skills of his physicians. He had a stroke several years ago which left his right side permanently weak. Several weeks ago one of his several physicians took him to surgery for a carotid endarterectomy, in which the narrowed artery to the brain is reamed clean to prevent another stroke. But shortly after surgery he had first a heart attack and then a bad stroke, caused by a clot released—instead of removed—in surgery.

He is very thin, very tall. He doesn't speak. When he rises at the beginning of the session he can barely stand, and quickly falls back into the wheelchair. But he is implacable and determined, utterly sure in spite of his silence of his surroundings and his purpose. Ten minutes later Custer Holland crosses the room with only a four-footed cane to assist him. His aide stands to the side, in silent, proud approval.

A woman slowly wheels in and turns her chair around in a corner, where she silently watches the proceedings with a mournful face. No one pays her any attention. She has lived in B Wing for years, with no medical orders for therapy. She has no medical diagnosis to justify the expense to the family, and neither insurance nor Medicare will pay for such vague gifts as increased flexibility, a parcel more of strength or endurance, the warmth of a small portion of individual attention. Individual attention isn't cheap. Like most patients who live in an intermediate-care facility (ICF), her doctor—whom she sees three or four times a year—has ordered "activity as tolerated," an open-ended and almost meaningless statement that gives the nurses and aides permission, but no mandate, to help the woman walk and exercise. They often haven't time; always the days are full of tasks that *have* been mandated. So several times a day she comes to the therapy room and waits, hoping one of the assistants can find a few extra minutes to walk with her. They try to accommodate her. But today Martin is scurrying the aides through the most vital treatments, hoping to send them home as soon as possible, worried about the weather. After half an hour of silent observation, the woman leaves.

Addie, one of the aides, watches a man in a wheelchair raise his leg parallel to the ground, then lower it again, fifteen times. The man's wife stands nearby, nervous, concerned. She catches Martin's eye as he walks past, and asks why the man complains of pain in his buttocks weeks after his hip surgery.

"It looks to me like he's got a positive gluteus medius weakness," Martin tells her, scrupulous with detail. "It takes time. They had to retract those muscles when they did the surgery." He looks at her expectantly.

After a pause and a blink the woman replies. "He's not a total loss, then?"

Stroke has a terrifying sound, with echoes of finality and demise, conjuring pictures of the inexorable movement of clock hands, oars slicing through water, the flogging of a whip. When it is the brain that is struck such a blow, nerves are buried in blood, choked blue from lack of oxygen, crushed by unexpected pressure. The damage is usually permanent, immediate, and sometimes bizarre in the extreme.

Anyone can have a stroke bestowed upon him, at any time.

A certain number of people walk the days of their lives with wispy, ballooning vessels in their brains, known as berry aneurysms, gently expanding with the rush of blood until they burst the way that a balloon, too full, bursts with a heart-stopping sound. A friend of mine, a cheerful and vigorous carpenter I'd known for over a decade, woke one morning with one side of his mouth drooling, the arm and leg on that side drooping uncontrollably. He was a lucky victim: several weeks later he was back to scampering on roofs, back to trivial conversations that had seemed so impossible when his tongue refused to obey. The bleeding hole in his brain had simply stopped, backed up, reversed itself. He may wake again one day, and find himself not himself, his body not his own. He tries not to think about it.

A much more common cause of stroke is a blood clot or bit of tissue that rides the stream into the brain, until it finds itself lodged in a tunnel too small. Stroke can be caused by many things; in its turn it causes shocking damage—and death. It is the third leading killer in the United States.

High blood pressure, or hypertension, carries with it a six-times-higher risk of a stroke than normal blood pressure. Half of all strokes happen to hypertensive people. Diabetes, obesity, smoking, alcoholism, even climate and the hardness of the water have been implicated in stroke. And age, which grants all these blessings and more, is perhaps the biggest risk factor of all: after the age of fifty-five, your risk of a stroke increases exponentially. At any given time, about twenty percent of the patients in Harvest Moon are there—either in the short run, for therapy, or in the long run, for life—because of strokes.

The aftermath, which one wakes to gradually, depends utterly on the site of the damage. The prognosis—your chances of returning to anything resembling what you were—depends on your age, your health, and, curiously, your personality. The ability to accept change and limits serves the stroke victim well. About a fourth of all stroke victims die from the first episode, some immediately, some months later. If progress is to be made, it must be made within six months; after that time, give or take the small kindnesses of steady therapy, the damage is permanent. This is the motive behind therapy schedules that seem almost frenetic at times to the worn and tired patient. In the end, about half of the survivors are severely disabled, and it is this, more than any other thing, that fills the word *stroke* with such power to frighten.

Irma Washington, a tall, fat, black woman, sits all day in a geriatric chair, a high-backed wheelchair with thick arms and a restraining table. Her big mouth hangs wide open, and she drools, the opening vulnerable and obscenely pink. Sometimes she moans. One arm is crooked in the classic posture of the stroke victim: elbow bent in half, wrist rotated inward, fingers clenched. She is fed by a tube in her nose, which is in its turn fed by a pump hooked on the back of her chair. There is something forgettable about Irma Washington—she is always the same, with an unchanging flatness in her face. She has been in this condition for nearly two years and could, it seems, go on for many more. Occasionally she smiles an infant smile for John Eldizondo, the nurse's aide. But her most human response is a sad one: she cries when Paula Schulz approaches with the toenail clippers.

When I walk the halls of Harvest Moon, when I recall patients in this and a half dozen other nursing homes, stroke is often what I am remembering. I see it in the postures, the arm held askew, the recalcitrant leg and foot bent inward, stubborn. I hear it in the voices, in Max's babble and Tillie Mott's blurred and retarded phrasings—and in Custer Holland's simple silence. I have seen so often that horrid sameness, the unchanging flat expression, and tried to look past it, underneath, for an explanation. My patients, these people so suddenly brought to ground, have refused to eat, claiming there is no food; demanded to walk, having no strength in their legs; grown incoherently enraged at my requests and limits. I am sure I have, as both a nurse and a curious passerby, failed to see what is, after all, so easy to miss: the odd and inexplicable symptoms of a stroke. These enigmatic clinical terms, mouthfuls of Latin roots—*stereognosis, graphesthesia, damaged proprioception*—come to startling, riveting life here.

Some strokes bear with them a kind of damage called *field cut*. In a field cut, one half of what is normally seen is gone. It simply disappears to the mind's eye. Field cut is often accompanied by an actual change in perceptual concepts, so that the angry woman who refuses to eat an invisible meal not only can't see the plate, she can't realize she cannot see it. It fails to *exist* for her. And is that so very odd, so rare? As I hurry down C Wing, late for an appointment, I see flashes of lives through doorways, still frames, caught moments frozen and lost. I see thin old men silently struggling to release the restraints that bind them, hear voices calling, calling with the same helpless, ceaseless words. These people suffer a refusal to accept what can't be seen, extending even to their own bodies, so that the arm and leg that hang in midair seem to belong to another person who has misplaced them. It is a kind of ultimate materialism. The stroke has damaged the brain in such a way that reality is literally misconceived; its victims truly don't know the nature of their illness, and by the nature of their illness *cannot* know it. I hurry to an appointment—which surely can't be so important—past scenes of astonishing poignancy, barely aware of the hungry lives buried there. I would like to understand this illness, these odd symptoms of delusion and inattention I suffer from, that cut away half or more of what I see. And by the nature of my illness I cannot know it.

Sophie Feldman has lived in Harvest Moon almost five years. She suffers a fate hard to justify, impossible to explain with any satisfaction. Mrs. Feldman, tall and broad and proud, had a thalamic stroke—that is, a stroke struck, discretely, her thalamus, the small essential portion of the brain buried deep in the interior. Thalamic strokes cause a peculiar and awful kind of damage to the brain: the almost constant awareness of intractable, incurable pain. The thalamus contains the neural equipment for appreciating many sensations: pain, temperature, touch, vibration, even part of the sensation of balance. The pain that results from damage to the thalamus is spontaneous, devilish, extreme. Mrs. Feldman's entire right side is almost constantly in agony, so searingly torturous that at times she faints from it. She has had relief from the pain only with doses of narcotics dangerously high; she is addicted to tranquilizers and mood elevators. I sit in the corner today and listen to the care team discuss, as they have discussed many times, ideas that might help her.

Martin King suggests acupuncture. Paula Schulz wonders if DMSO, dimethyl sulfoxide, might help. DMSO sometimes relieves arthritis pain. Charlene Parrott has heard rumors about new laser surgery to the thalamus itself. Paula mentions, reluctantly, the possibility of a sympathectomy, a drastic surgery of last resort which would slice all the nerves to the affected side, leaving it completely numb.

Sophie Feldman's only relative is her son, who pays for all her care. He is very conservative about her treatment, rejects the notion—and the costs—of "quack cures" like acupuncture.

"We might start planting the seeds in Sophie's mind," suggests Paula. "She'll tell him. Acupuncture's safe, there's no side effects, and if it reduces her pain by even one-tenth, what an improvement in her quality of life that would be. It's certainly worth pursuing."

Everyone agrees. Paula will casually discuss it with Sophie. Eventually, diplomatically, she will approach the son. Charlene Parrott puts her head on her forearms and peers up at the faces around her.

"*I've* been here five years, and all we've ever talked about for Sophie is her pain," she says, not expecting any comment.

Such a grim picture is only partially true. There are many successes. Harvest Moon, with its emphasis on rehabilitation, admits so many stroke victims that the staff has become quite adept in their care. And though half of the stroke patients remain seriously disabled, the other half eventually progress to an independence in daily tasks. While they may never be able to live alone again—although many do—they can walk, dress and feed themselves, and often cook their own meals. And their minds are clear and free of confusion.

Annie Brun paid sympathy visits to her daughter's mother-in-law, a "shirttail relative," who had had a stroke and was in Harvest Moon for therapy. But two weeks after the visits started, Annie herself had a stroke. "I had guests, and when I got up to get refreshments, I noticed I was a little wobbly. And it got worse."

Annie suffered right hemiplegia, a paralysis of the right arm and leg caused by a stroke in the left side of the brain. Hemiplegia is a classic and very common symptom of stroke, and is usually accompanied by both spastic tremors in the muscles—sudden and uncontrollable trembling—and weak flaccidity of the same muscles. The weak side is unbalanced and often painful, and anxiety makes the tremors worse. Annie Brun was lucky; she had no other complications, no loss of language, no confusion or personality changes. She faced only the simple task of learning to walk and dress and feed herself again. A few days after her stroke, she was discharged from the hospital and admitted to Harvest Moon, a few doors down the hall from her relative.

"I thought I'd be over here two weeks and then be home," she says. "I didn't know what I was in for." A few weeks after her admission, competing with her friend in physical therapy, she seemed destined for a rapid recovery, but in early November Annie strained her hamstring. She had been able to walk sixty feet with a walker until then, but for almost two weeks could only go a few steps. Her second recovery has been fast and, in a way, almost pleasant for Annie. It is an adventure of sorts, a change of pace, to be out of her home and in a charged and busy place. She is never bored, happily watches "Wheel of

Fortune" and "Jeopardy" every day, goes to physical therapy twice a day and occupational therapy every afternoon, reads, and chats. She watches with a detached interest the people around her.

"After I first went here, there was a sweet person in my room who couldn't talk. Her speech was affected. I introduced myself and she pointed to her mouth and I knew she couldn't talk, but that was okay because I talked enough for both of us. Then they moved her out and brought in Bernice, who had had a hip replacement. We've having a ball!" She pauses in her verbosity. "It's been four of the most fun weeks I've had in a long time."

Aphasia is the oddest of all stroke's scars, the most disconcerting. It silences when one most desires company, walls a person, freshly wounded, into a world in which he or she is the sole inhabitant. Aphasia steals language, both that which is given and that which is received, a gift of remarkable value, from others. It severs its victims from the most fundamental events of society. Aphasia is Max Kleiner's trademark, his signature, his shibboleth in a tribe of one.

Aphasia is a disorder of processing caused by the brain damage. It affects the ability to receive, understand, and use language, and affects every effort the patient might make toward some kind of recovery. The nurses, the physical therapist, family members—every person the patient comes in contact with is presented with a wall of wordlessness. The wall may be made of words, of chants, of vowel sounds, of real words—but the effect is of no words at all.

At Harvest Moon most of the weight of therapy for aphasia falls on Barb Coulter, the part-time speech and language pathologist. She is a neat, quiet, pretty woman, with curly light blond hair and pale skin, pink-cheeked and blue-eyed. She wears large, clear glasses, conservative, plain clothes. She had

79

planned to become a mathematician before she flunked out of calculus.

Her first approach with victims of aphasia is to figure out, as closely as possible, where the main problem lies. "Sometimes just reading the history will help, knowing where the stroke was," she says. "There are tests all over the place we use to try to pinpoint the problems. Then you take it from there. Sometimes drill work is effective and sometimes it's not. You try something, and give it a good shot, and if it doesn't work, then you have to change your program."

If a person cannot speak, or can't speak coherently, how can you test for confusion or memory loss? Rarely is aphasia a "pure" symptom. Problems with processing buried deep in the brain are mixed with weakened tongue and throat muscles, shortened attention spans, impulsiveness, personality changes, and intellectual losses. They are all slippery eels of bruised neurons and dead cells, devilish, passing strange.

But aphasia is rarely silent. More often it is noisy and meaningless, and marked by perseverance and a bewitched loquaciousness. I have met—and heard unseen—so many different people calling "Help me, help me, help me," endlessly, dully, hopelessly, but always in desperation, that I've come to think of it as a moral of some kind, a patterned response and a reasonable one to a terrible, permanent imprisonment.

How long does one struggle with a world full of nonsense, uncontrolled jungle chatter, farrago and twaddle, before one is legitimately insane? Max Kleiner might have come to his stroke sure and confident and rich of mind, might even have left his stroke with that mind intact, but I suspect it curled up some time past for a long, long nap. He seems happy enough, with whatever we have to measure happiness—smiles, roving eyes, a free touch, and, of course, talk. He does talk.

Barb spends more time working with dysarthria and apraxia than aphasia. There is more that can be done with the first two. Dysarthria is a defect of muscle movement, so that you cannot make your lips form words, cannot make your tongue move. The victim must struggle and concentrate, forcing the stubborn muscles of the tongue and lips and throat into a set, learned pattern in order to speak. The patient must often overcompensate, learn a whole new exaggerated manner of speech. "It's like trying to lift a six-hundred-pound weight. If you're not strong enough, you *just can't do it.*" She teaches exercise and concentration, and some patients achieve success— at mumbling, blurred, but comprehensible speech.

Apraxia is less readily defined and harder to treat; its manifestations slide in and around those of aphasia. Apraxia is a kind of canyon with the bridge washed out; its victim is clearheaded and knows exactly what he wants to say with his perfectly intact tongue and lips—but he can't make them move. The connection—the *translation*—of thought into action is broken. In a similar way the stroke victim looks at his paralyzed leg and wills it to straighten, strains *in his mind* as though lifting a great weight—and nothing happens. I can almost sense this: I look at my left index finger and order it to move, just a little, to the side, but at the same time I order my finger to ignore my orders. I can feel a struggle take place, a strangely uncomfortable struggle. Very soon I quit, and allow the finger a small motion, a compensation, and the relief is enormous.

But all these demons are just exotica for Barb, interesting breaks from the repetitive labor of teaching people to swallow again. A dysphagic patient chokes: the unconscious choreography of the throat, slipping air down one tube and food down another a short distance away, fails. With trial and error Barb can sometimes find certain foods—or certain textures—that a person can tolerate, like thick purees such as applesauce. A stroke can leave a person permanently dependent on nursing care for several reasons, such as being unable to walk, or being confused. But the loss of the ability to swallow is the trickiest one of all, for such a person not only requires nursing care of some kind but must be fed artificially. Like the wheelchair, the feeding tube is a giant obstacle in the return to normal life.

Every four or five months, Barb Coulter and Paula Schulz,

81

the nurse practitioner, decide to pull out Irma Washington's feeding tube. Irma in her fat black blankness will suddenly come "a little bit more alive," as Barb puts it, and with the consent of family and physician the tube is removed. Then Barb visits daily, trying a bit of this and that, a taste here, a swallow there, and watches the result with rapt attention. For a few days Irma seems to get it, will strain to slide the food where it belongs. But she always slips away again, into that empty place she so long has inhabited, and chokes, and Paula sadly orders the tube to go down again.

Barb likes the little gains of her work, the problem solving, the creativity required. "We really do a lot of exploring, and sometimes there is only one thing that will work with a patient. You have to do a lot of work to figure out what it is. With this population the steps are small. You don't see overnight successes very often. But if you work with somebody for two or three months and eventually they are able to go someplace a little more independent, where they are going to be comfortable, then it's worth it."

Barb is thirty-one—"it sounds old but it doesn't feel old"— and one of the changes she has experienced at Harvest Moon is an appreciation of age. "I look at people who are sixty and they are not as old as they used to be. Sixty used to be just forever, really old. You have a lot of options—you can be a little shriveled up old person, or you can be one of the ones that are happy and have accepted their age."

While a person waits through the days, ticking off hours between therapy and the rest it requires, boredom is ever-present. It breathes down the neck, perches on the bedclothes. And when therapy fails, when its simple progressions are progress enough, boredom—of a different kind for the confused, a tedium, a going on—again comes to roost. Margery Todd is in charge of the activity department, which includes two part-time assistants. She arranges everything from a wildly successful ceramics program to dog shows and church services, as well as visiting each "isolated" patient—patients who are bedridden or unable or unwilling to socialize in groups—at least weekly.

"Loneliness is something I see a lot. I see myself spending more time with the patients who don't really have anybody, have no children. I find myself spending maybe an extra five or ten minutes a day with them." She is a big and bright woman in her early thirties, heavy and strong, with eyes deeply outlined and shadowed and cheeks red with blusher. Around her neck she wears a cross decorated with tiny rubies.

"I don't think the patients need a lot of fillers, unimportant things to be doing throughout the day. They need a feeling of accomplishment. They need a feeling of doing something for someone else, being involved in the world. I think a lot of the time they're overlooked, their opinions are not requested." Margery has developed an involved ceramics program, in which patients make vases, plates, cups, saucers, and more throughout the year. The items are fired in a kiln and then the patients paint them, and at Christmas sell their handiwork— always successfully—to staff and family members. The money raised is spent on parties and field trips later on.

Trivial Pursuit was Margery's idea, too. "It's been really popular," she notes. "And they do extremely well. And there again I think a lot of people don't ask them questions about history or things about music, and it might just take one question to bring back a lot of memories. Bingo is real popular, too, and they play for money. They win a quarter a game. There is competition. And it's great number identification, eye-hand coordination, not just something to sit and pass the time of day. We have seen incredible success with patients that had strokes, who at first couldn't identify numbers."

Card games, too: I watched Cathy Bosley, one of Margery's assistants, lead a group through a game of blackjack. She walked around the table, bending over each person's hand, explaining in a stage whisper how many points they held, advising them to hold or take a card. She had to beg for bets: "Bertha! Can you place your bet now?" she yelled in a fat woman's ear, until Bertha grumpily pushed a chip forward. Flora stayed, Sophie Feldman asked to be hit twice, Verna folded, and Buddy, always the gambler, went broke asking for more and more cards. At last she came to Tillie Mott, her hand huddled in her lap, loose. Cathy looked suddenly startled. "She got a twenty-one!" she cried, in real surprise. "I don't believe this. She got a twenty-one!" Cathy paid sleeping Tillie her chips, reluctantly, I thought.

"A lot of my friends say, 'How can you do that, that kind of thing?' " says Margery. "But I think in a lot of ways these people have taught me that it's going to be okay. I don't worry about getting old now. But I have found over the years that I've put more distance in my relationships with the patients. It hurts to lose fifty grandmas and grandpas."

Margery is a confidante to some of the people she visits privately. For some she is their only visitor except for the nurses. "I'm fortunate enough to be able to spend a lot of one-on-one time with them. I think at times they find nursing a little bit threatening, and if they have a problem they're afraid to say anything, that there might be retaliation. We try to look for constructive solutions that will help." She shifts in the chair, gathers together the leftovers of her hurried, talked-through lunch. Margery has worked here six years. She recently married a man with several children, and knows that soon she'll have to quit this job. "I've asked myself a lot why I've stayed this long," she says. "I feel that in some way the patients are all right with me: that I am here and they are safe because I'm here."

CHAPTER SEVEN

Criteria

The Medicare system is full of backwaters and impediments, described in long columns of entangled lingo and code words. The regulations hold two themes especially dear: first, that these rules and explanations are lucid and clear, that there is nothing vague, no area for disagreement. The second theme of Medicare, strengthened a few years ago as the main thrust of Medicare's brave new future, is that every person is the same. This is a blank and blanket assumption: that every patient with the same diagnosis will suffer and recover in the same way and in the *same period of time*. It is a very strange assumption, utterly insupportable, and contrary to the most basic understanding of health and illness.

One of the most common injuries of the elderly is a fractured hip, product of weakening bones and fragile posture. According to Medicare, a sixty-six-year-old woman in good health who walks two miles a day, slips on an icy sidewalk, and breaks a hip, will recover in a certain period of time. Her care should cost, according to Medicare, a certain amount and no more. And that amount is all Medicare will pay. When an eighty-five-year-old man with a heart condition, diabetes, and mild confusion falls in his bathroom and breaks his hip (perhaps straining his shoulder in the process), Medicare will give him the same amount of time and pay the same amount of money for his care as the woman nearly two decades younger.

It is mid-December, and Martin King is teaching—as he has taught several times before, for the subject is never obsolete—a short seminar on how to position patients with hip fractures or hip replacements. He will teach it three times today. Martin has decided to grow a beard, to give himself a rougher look, but even with the short, ragged growth of four days on his chin he doesn't look scruffy. It isn't in his nature to look scruffy.

He is testing the table in the conference room for its strength; to properly demonstrate, he needs a prone subject. He leans against the table tentatively and feels it give, then looks at a quiet, attractive young woman nearby. She is a physical therapy student observing Martin's techniques. "You have insurance, don't you?" he asks, and invites her to be his model.

People with broken hips—either pinned for repair or replaced with steel—are the second biggest group at Harvest Moon, behind strokes. An elderly person can fracture a hip—the bones grow brittle and thin with age—in a fall before they hit the ground. The torque of twisting to avoid the abrupt landing can itself split the bone into pieces. Some hips shatter as though made of glass, splinter like smashed wood; some, like Anna Rosenbaum's, have so little fabric left that the rags cannot be sewn together. Paula suspects that Margaret Bond faces this in her innocent optimism: "Her bones are full of holes," she says in her bluntness. So Margaret waits in her room, paying out dearly saved hundreds of dollars a week, waiting, probably in vain, for her hips to tolerate a fraction of her weight. Because Medicare regulations reflect a world where every fractured hip is the same, there is no room for such a hiatus, no money, no time. Margaret has only so long to recover, and so she saves her days, her precious Medicare days, for the possibility of renewal—and more expensive treatment—in the future. In a sense she is on vacation from her own rehabilitation, which Medicare claims should be a straightforward and predictable journey. She waits on a side road until she is well enough to travel further. It is this common problem that Barb Coulter referred to when she said, shaking her head, "It's got me into financial planning for when *I'm* eighty years old. I've learned a lot about Medicare and what happens to your money when you get old."

Martin rolls the silent, blank-faced girl back and forth across the table, talking as he does of the many restrictions laid on the patient with a fractured or implanted hip. It used to be standard practice to confine such patients to bed for weeks; as a result of the forced inaction, people quickly developed pneumonia, bedsores, thrombophlebitis (which can lead to, among other things, thrombic strokes), atrophied muscles, and even weaker bones. Now people are pulled from bed the day after surgery, first to stand, then to walk—and walk and walk. A person with a pinned hip must learn, now and forever, to avoid twisting. Even the slight bend of a reach behind one's shoulder can pop a pin from position. Martin demonstrates the many positions to be avoided, the few to be encouraged, propping his assistant's complacent legs with pillows fore and behind. In his mild and unassuming voice, he lists the taboos: crossing the knees, flexing a hip past a spare 90 degrees, overstuffed chairs, low chairs, squatting, toilets without raised seats. And all this is for naught if the patient falls again.

From its origins in the casual philanthropy of politicians, Medicare has become too full of its own good, zealous in pursuit of the proper. It is a tentacle in the mutation of public policy called Social Security, with tentacles of its own. Medicare is legislated by the Social Security Act, but managed separately under the Health Care and Financing Administration, or HCFA. (Employees of HCFA, which they call "Hic-faa," like a mild belch, are defensive about this last point. "Medicare is *equal* to Social Security," one senior administrator told me huffily.)

Few people—even senior administrators—claim to understand more than a part of Medicare or Social Security any more. Workers in the system function within small areas of expertise, able to explain only one or two threads of the running tapestry. Administrative phone numbers aren't published; inquiries must pass through branch after branch of front-line receptionists and assistants, and referrals are often accompanied by the pained voice of uncertainty. Studies have shown that workers will answer the same question—hard, factual questions, yes-no questions—differently from day to day, depending on how it is phrased and who is doing the asking.

Perhaps it is just me, but I doubt it. Even with the law in front of me I'm not sure what the rules are. In subpart G, subsection 405.702 of the Medicare rules on payment—because there is never a guarantee that Medicare will pay any bill—is the description of the "Notice of Initial Determination." It reads: "After a request for payment under Part A of Title XVIII of the Act is filed with the intermediary by or on behalf of the individual who received . . . services, and the intermediary has ascertained whether the items and services are covered under Part A of Title XVIII, and where appropriate, ascertained and made payments of amounts due or has ascertained that no payments were due (see subsection 405.401(c)) . . ." Well, that's when I start skimming. Any approach to the bounty of Medicare costs the consumer, as well as the providers, aggravation and bewilderment.

I know I'm not alone in this. A judge, in exasperation, wrote: "As program after program has evolved, there has developed a degree of complexity in the Social Security Act and particularly the regulations which makes them almost unintelligible to the uninitiated. There should be no such form of reference as '45 C.F.R.[sec] 248.3 (c) (1) (ii) (B) (2)'; a draftsman who has gotten himself into a position requiring anything like this should make a fresh start."

Fresh starts, however, are not something the federal government excels in. Medicare regulations are constantly changing, constantly being refined or mauled depending on your point of view, and by the time the consequences of any one change in policy are visible, a new change is already on the books. Like the tax laws they are regulations of opinion, dependent on the fluid interpretations of words like "reasonable" and "generally" and "appropriate" by people who read case studies, match them to protocol and subsections, and never meet the people involved. They are subject to a very human capriciousness that may be inevitable in a system that attempts to provide altruism on a budget.

From any point of view, Medicare is radically misunderstood. Many people think of it as a free and comprehensive insurance policy for their years after 65, one that provides simple—and complete—coverage for their medical needs. The truth is far different.

Medicare is a complex and changing insurance system, available to Social Security recipients—but not automatically, you must apply for it—and to certain classes of disabled people under sixty-five. There are two parts, hospital coverage and medical coverage, which pay for different services, cost different amounts, and are subject to different interpretations. Premiums for these two separate policies run from a few dollars a month to nearly $200 a month. Premiums must be renewed at certain intervals—and if you fail to apply at certain times, or renew at certain times, you must wait months for coverage to begin. Each kind of care—office visits, physical therapy, hospital care, nursing home care, drugs, wheelchairs, home nursing—is paid in different amounts, for different periods of time. There are significantly varying deductibles, too, and they are big: for any hospitalization under sixty days, the first $400 is not paid. For hospitalizations over sixty days, the first $100 a *day* is not paid. Medicare pays in benefit periods that vary according to the kind of care received and where it is received. And all these exceptions and omissions are the responsibility of the patient.

A lot of Medicare recipients will never have to worry about these hindrances. Only a small fraction of people stay in a hospital more than sixty days. But for that group, two points are relevant: $100 a day adds up very quickly; and a fair number of people who are that sick, whose recovery is that slow, are going to end up in nursing homes. Salesmen for so-called Medigap insurance, private policies which purport to fill in, at a cost, these holes, report difficulty selling their product not because of the price, but because people honestly don't believe Medicare has holes. And it is nursing home care that is the biggest hole, and possibly the biggest misunderstanding.

"A lot of people think that if you need nursing home care you automatically are skilled and should get Medicare. We have a terrible time making people understand that long-term care is not extended care," says Paula Schulz. *Long-term care* refers to intermediate- or ICF-level care—basic, usually permanent, care for people like the unresponsive, shuffling Cecil Lunt. Medicare will not pay for *any* such care, *ever*. It is solely directed toward care that may have some foreseeable "benefit" in terms of progress or rehabilitation. Such care is called *extended care,* an extension of the hospital, and is what is offered in the skilled wing of Harvest Moon.

The most recent changes in Medicare regulation have taken the idea of rehabilitation even further, to the point of classifying all illnesses in categories of cost. The regulations, called the Diagnostic Related Groups, or DRGs, set an amount of money to be paid, in advance, to institutions providing care. Each diagnosis—and a patient is allowed only one DRG per admission, regardless of the true number of illnesses he may suffer—is worth a certain amount of money. Regardless of the person's condition, no more money will be forthcoming. Physicians have been openly encouraged by hospitals to discharge patients earlier than was previously done in order to keep the hospital from losing money on sicker patients. One result is the surge in skilled nursing facilities, often the only reasonable place for such patients to go—many are too sick to go home. Within this skilled setting, with an appropriate diagnosis that meets the essential criteria—potential for rehabilitation, requiring skilled nursing and therapy, and care that is both "reasonable and necessary"—a person's bills might be paid for by Medicare: *part* of the bills, that is, for a limited period of time, as long as the patient has been hospitalized for at least three days in a row, not counting the day of discharge, and is admitted to the skilled facility within thirty days of leaving the hospital. This specific situation is the only time Medicare will pay for nursing home care.

In general, skilled care is that which requires round-the-clock supervision of a licensed nurse—usually a registered nurse. The person's needs must be too complex, too unpredictable, or too serious to be left to aides or practical nurses alone. Medicare has devised special conditions and procedures that qualify as skilled care: daily teaching to develop independence in care; training to regain control of bladder or bowel; care for fractured bones or unhealed wounds, for healing of serious bedsores, for a healing colostomy, after complicated tracheotomies or other airway problems; conditions requiring use of feeding tubes for drainage or medication, injections, or intravenous lines. Less commonly, skilled care can mean the complicated judgments and flexible approach required to care for people with erratic or unstable behavior, or with unusually complex and varying medical conditions. To qualify a patient under this last criterion requires a concerted involvement of the entire rehabilitation team.

Such a list would seem to encompass a great many things, but it does not. Each criterion is heavily weighted with the demand that it lead within a period of time to improvement. The words *predictable, necessary, reasonable, restorative, progress,* and *stability* occur again and again. A pamphlet given to Medicare recipients to explain the benefits says, for example, that Medicare won't pay if you visit your doctor "more often than is the usual medical practice in your area," or stay in a hospital or skilled facility "longer than you need to be there." The censure is clear. One must show constant motion to qualify, and the decision lies not with the patient, nurse, physician, or facility, but with Medicare.

The nurses must document not only the care they give, but the reason for providing skilled nursing care, every day, every shift. If a person is considered a skilled-care patient because they have a nasogastric feeding tube and will, it is hoped, learn to eat again, then every shift the nurses must note the placement of the NG tube, the number of times it is used, whether or not oral feedings are offered, and how both oral and tube feedings are tolerated. She must also write in her notes—and she writes one for each of her fifteen to twenty patients every day—about the person's activities, their mental state, their routine, their bowel and bladder, the condition of their skin, whether they have worn restraints, whether they show signs of any medical problems, such as a fever, in what ways they are limited in caring for themselves, if any teaching was done and how it was received, and whether the goals in the care plan are being met.

One part of Medicare pays the cost of nursing care, drugs, equipment, and rehabilitation therapy—but not doctor's services—for the first twenty days of a stay in a skilled facility. For the twenty-first through the hundredth day, it pays all but $50 a day. After one hundred days, it pays nothing. There are no extensions. To qualify for a new hundred-day benefit period, the patient must leave the facility and be gone for sixty days, and not receive any hospital or skilled nursing home care in that time. This is the bind Margaret Bond is in, with her hip that refuses to heal. Because she can't leave for home, and can't go forward with her therapy, "saving days" is her only choice. She does it because the cost of the skilled wing and the therapy she still expects in the future is more expensive than the out-of-pocket expenses she and her husband pay to keep her where she is.

Behind all these complex rules is something called the "waiver of liability," a very complex and fluid set of regulations freeing both individual patients and the facilities that provide care from the liability of costs *even* when the parties involved misinterpret Medicare law. In a sense the waiver of liability is a huge acknowledgment of how impossible it is to fully understand the system: it provides a way out for people who simply can't figure out whether a particular set of circumstances applies, whether particular treatments of specific combinations of conditions fit the criteria. It presupposes good intent as it bows to the inevitable, full of hems and haws and exceptions. The waiver of liability allows facilities to make a small fraction of "mistakes" in their interpretation of who and what is eligible for Medicare. Harvest Moon has a "denial rate" of about 2.4 percent—that is, about that many of its Medicare claims are considered inappropriate or ineligible by the Medicare reviewers, either because of the kind of treatment given or the nature of the illness. (Denials are often based on one of two problems: failure to progress, and a stay beyond "reasonable and necessary.") As long as the denial rates stay this low, Medicare will go ahead and pay for these inappropriate claims, and the patient himself will usually not know there was ever a concern. Each quarter-year Medicare begins tabulating the denial rate again; each quarter-year the slate is clean. And any time Medicare decides the denial rate is too high, or the denied claims raise the slightest suspicion, Medicare can refuse to guarantee payment for *any* Medicare claim in that facility.

Several months ago, in an almost whimsical about-face, Medicare canceled the entire waiver-of-liability clause. It was a blanket decision and wholly unexpected by people like Paula Schulz, whose job entails constant attempts to interpret and explain the Medicare requirements. With the waiver of liability removed, Harvest Moon had no expectation that Medicare would pay any bill, no pressure to bring to bear, no string to pull, no contract to wave. Suddenly every Medicare patient in the facility was a potential loss of thousands of dollars—after the fact. Paula, like a lot of other people in similar positions, made a lot of noise, and a month later the waiver was reinstated. But it left Paula shaken, reminded of the alien and unpredictable nature of the system, and of the difficulty, when approaching it, of even finding the front door.

One requirement of Medicare is that the facility establish a utilization review committee, or URC, to regularly review questionable cases and decide, before the claim comes to Medicare, whether the patient really qualifies for coverage. The URC can itself advise Harvest Moon to, in turn, advise a patient or the patient's family that his care no longer qualifies—or never qualified—for Medicare. Then the decision—to stay and pay, or to go—is up to the family, which has seventy-two hours to decide.

In day-to-day practice, the URC—which is a small group of people all part of or close to Harvest Moon—and the safety net of the waiver of liability allow the facility a certain amount of freedom in making decisions. Paula Schulz can, as long as the denial rate stays low, edge a few questionable cases through, take a small risk in order to keep a patient a week longer than absolutely necessary. She considers it a pleasant challenge.

Although the HCFA system manages Medicare, the actual distribution of money and assortment of claims is done by "third-party payors," or administrators. These are large insurance companies that bid for the right to handle Medicare claims in their area. The choices are limited; in Harvest Moon's metropolitan area of over a million in population, there are only two Medicare payors. Harvest Moon has chosen to use Blue Cross.

"I never get to talk to Medicare," groans Paula. "Who's Medicare?" She imitates the voice on the phone when she calls the Medicare offices; it is a weird and shrill monotone, the voice of an irritated robot. "Well, you know what the three criteria are, do they meet the three criteria, if they meet the three criteria then they are skilled, if they do not then they are not,

94

why are you bothering us?" She returns to her normal voice. "That's how they are. It's like there's this Medicare monster. Then there's this Blue Cross monster, too, who blames Medicare for everything, when indeed it is them and their doctors. If you ask Blue Cross who denies you, they say it's Medicare. But if you call Medicare, they deny *that*. You say, 'Who is Medicare, who denied this?' 'Well, our doctor, it's our doctor.' Who's the doctor?" Paula shakes her head.

"There's no humanitarianism in the rules," she continues. "If you stick a tube down someone's nose, they're skilled. If you feed him and plead with him and coax him to eat and watch his nutrition and watch his hydration, which takes ten times as long as dumping formula down a tube, then he's not skilled." Since without Medicare many people must turn to welfare, it is in the interest of a facility to keep a person on a tube as long as possible, to actually *discourage* the progress Medicare demands until it threatens to stop payment for lack of it. Medicare is not concerned with the ultimate fate of any one person—or even of a population—but with how its funds are used in the immediate present. If a person is almost, but not quite, ready to return home but a benefit period is over, Medicare will stop payment. Sometimes the patient or his family will decide to go ahead with a discharge, sometimes a facility—hospital or nursing home—will subtly or not subtly encourage it. The same person may return to the hospital a week later, sicker than ever—perhaps with a newly broken hip from a fall unlikely to have happened under nursing care. Several recent studies have begun to examine, individually, the several thousand cases in which people were discharged from a hospital and rehospitalized for the same problem less than a week later. (This doesn't always have to be bad medicine: a hip surgeon tells me that, though he would prefer to do repairs or replacements of both hips in the same patient at the same time, thereby saving both himself and the patient time, expense, and pain, Medicare will only pay for one hip at a time. So he does each hip separately, in separate hospitalizations.) It is not an efficient system, and not a thrifty one, and always the patient is the x in a bouncing equation, treated to new rounds of treatment and waiting.

The Diagnostic Related Groups, or DRGs, are the heart of the matter now. They rule Medicare. There are 470 diagnoses in the DRGs, and they classify every mishap that can befall the human body. Each diagnosis is weighted, and each weight reflects a cost—or price—that is an estimate of the average cost of providing care for that diagnosis in a certain geographical area. Medicare pays for only one diagnosis at a time. A staff member from the Special Committee on Aging, partly responsible for the DRGs, said about the idea, "What we expected was for hospitals to make money on half the patients and lose money on the other." The detailed permutations of this truly incredible system have been dealt with in detail elsewhere. But the idea that large for-profit corporations would voluntarily lose money on half of a commodity out of kindness is truly a wonder. The DRG system has created instead distasteful incentive programs that encourage physicians to discharge patients when their money runs out, regardless of the patients' conditions. A California hospital has offered to split the savings with the physician when a patient is discharged before the money runs out. Another ploy is to discharge a patient and readmit him under a different diagnosis, for a new benefit period. The different weights are made use of, too: angina, a kind of chest pain caused by low oxygen levels in the heart muscle, is a lower weight than "chest pain" or "possible heart attack"; consequently, many physicians no longer diagnose angina in their patients. Each is granted a possible heart attack.

But not every worse-than-average patient can be sent home from the hospital. This has proved to be a boon of a kind to the skilled facilities like Harvest Moon. The number and variety of patients being admitted is growing rapidly, and their stays are shorter. Over the last two weeks on C Wing, four people died soon after they were admitted: one after nine days, another in six days, another in four days, and the fourth person died in only two days. Such rapid turnover, as it were, was unheard-of five years ago, and so were the complexities required for their care. The skilled wing of Harvest Moon now boasts medical problems and treatments even more varied than an average hospital ward. In extended care there are no specialties but perseverance.

"It's too much, just too much," says Bonnie Pereira. After four years she wonders how much more she can take. "I guess they think if you can organize yourself and set your priorities, you'll get it all done. But it's just too much. I don't like leaving things undone, and I have to now. I never had to do that before."

"It's made life incredibly more difficult here. The patients are a lot tougher," says Erin Myers, a nurse on the evening shift for five years. "Sometimes I think they put a hook out on the street and grab whoever goes by, particularly if they have a tube." She grunts in bitter amusement.

For all its demands, Medicare still pays only a small portion of annual nursing home costs in the United States—less than five percent. Medicaid, the federal program that pays for health care for poor people, is responsible for paying for over half of all nursing home costs in the country.

Like its sister, Medicaid is labyrinthine and fluid, fettered by a complicated bureaucracy of hands working independently of each other. Many of the standards used by Medicaid, such as the differentiation between intermediate and skilled care, are borrowed from Medicare. For the many thousands of people who can't qualify for Medicare because of age or condition, the only alternative is insolvency and a permanent dependence on welfare. People like Buddy Mullin, the young accident victim whose family no longer visits, and Howie Kramer, who has almost no family at all, will spend the rest of their lives supported by Medicaid. People like Max Kleiner, who are old enough to qualify but whose "potential for rehabilitation" is nonexistent, are in the same position. Medicare will pay nothing, insurance policies pay for long-term care very rarely, and few families have the resources to support a relative for years. These thousands of people have literally no one to take care of them, except for all of us together.

Howie Kramer and Buddy Mullin are both labeled "heavy cost," a heady and cumbrous title that reflects their intimate needs accurately, if rather coldly. Neither has family or money, neither can expect a future very different from the present. They share a room and are strangers to each other. Buddy's bed is covered with a pretty spread, the walls with posters and stereo equipment and stuffed animals. In contrast, Howie's small space is empty and bare, the walls broken only by an old, small photograph of his daughter and a calendar. Buddy has visitors all day long, and recently spent a weekend at a bowling tournament for disabled people. A group of motorcycle enthusiasts have given Buddy a remote-controlled toy motorcycle for racing in the parking lot. Howie is—well, Howie is just Howie, mostly alone, usually lonely, avoiding and, more and more, avoided.

He has decided he will eat only buttermilk now. All day, he refuses the food brought to him and demands buttermilk. Each of his visitors is asked to bring him a glass of buttermilk, and he asks me when I arrive, before we say hello. "It's in the fridge," he tells me airily, and sure enough, there is a quart of it there, with his name on it. I pour him a glass and hold it, straw bent, so he can drink. He slurps it up in one long and noisy gulp.

Howie is upset about his radio, the big tabletop model bought years ago. "My mother bought this dear old radio," he says. It is tuned perpetually to a beautiful music station. "She told me it cost almost a hunnerd-an-fordy dollars." His persecuted anxiety returns; the calm of receiving his buttermilk is already fading. "I don't know if that's true or not. Sometimes it doesn't work very well."

CHAPTER EIGHT

Perpetual Motion

A pile of charts balances precariously on the table as team conference begins. Eyes wander to the window and its shafts of sunny, incongruous light.

Nancy Rice is making a last bid for more intensive therapy with a dying man.

"His eyes are so bright. It seems we should give it a shot," she says, almost wistfully, and glances around the table. "Am I out of line here?"

"Yes," answers Charlene Parrott, not attempting to hide a smile.

Paula scribbles, apparently not listening, then looks up so abruptly everyone turns to her. She looks at Nancy.

"We want him to be mobile when he dies, right?"

No one answers, his chart is closed, the discussion proceeds to the next name on the list, Conrad Berry.

In late September Conrad Berry, an active man in his early eighties, had a heart attack followed several hours later by a severe stroke. He fell, as tall, lean men fall, from a wealth of independence to a bed from which he will never rise. But he stubbornly refused to die when the doctors told his grieving daughter he would, and instead, spurred by the efforts of his physicians, he came to a kind of equipoise—a balance. For almost three months he has been a patient at Harvest Moon, fed by a tube which must be replaced several times a week. He pulls it out, again and again, and so his hands must be tied to the bedrails with soft cloth restraints. He cannot control bowel or bladder, is paralyzed on one side, has lost most of his vision, and can talk only in the globular murmurings of the aphasic.

"It doesn't look like he's ready to do much for himself yet," says Charlene, with a slight bite of sarcasm in her voice.

Barb Coulter talks about her work with Mr. Berry. She has managed to improve his swallowing, with considerable effort, so much so that he can swallow thick liquids now. But he can't coordinate his swallowing with his breathing, and becomes upset and frightened when food is placed in his mouth.

"He has a heck of a bite reflex and he's not very cooperative," she adds, explaining that she's told him he must choose either food or the tube. "I'm not *real* sure I can explain the relationship to him."

"His Medicare is about to exhaust," Paula points out. Nancy adds, almost as an afterthought, that Mr. Berry's daughter is still hoping to find his Living Will, signed over a year ago and now lost.

"He wanted to go, go, go every day. He had a girlfriend. He just couldn't stand to stay home; every day we were always going someplace."

Conrad Berry's daughter, Patricia Miller, is a passive, worn woman. She huddles in her coat and speaks in flat, tired tones. Her father's illness has shocked her into inertness. Her hair, eyes, skin all have the dullness of depression. She visits him every day—sometimes two and three times a day, hating the time at his bedside and unable to stay away.

"I just have to see how he's doing. There's just a lot of

things they can't take care of, they can't go in there twenty-four hours a day and watch. It does cost a lot of money but you have to understand." She speaks slowly, looking at her hands held tightly together on the table in front of her. "Oh, it depresses me, seeing those people in the hall like my dad. People just sitting there with a tube in their nose, not moving. He doesn't think anybody should live like this. He always said that. He didn't plan it this way." Conrad Berry refused to visit friends and relatives in nursing homes, proclaiming out loud that people should not be kept alive like "vegetables," that nursing homes were "warehouses." Patricia was given only two days' warning from the hospital that he would be discharged, and had no time—and no strength—to look at different homes and choose with care. She picked Harvest Moon on the recommendation of the hospital social worker, never expecting her father to live for months—to live, apparently, for many months more.

"I'm just hoping that he won't go on living, living like this, because it isn't the way he wanted to be. It seems funny. He's just like a baby now."

The team discusses Anna Rosenbaum for a few minutes. Her hip infection hasn't improved. Martin King says, "She's quite a fighter, that's the way she is." But her fight won't heal her hip. He holds little hope for her ever walking again.

"Wanna maximize her?" asks Nancy, using the all-purpose term for therapy that may yield only small results. The team tries to "maximize level of functioning"—that is, to do what they can, hope for the best.

"Sometimes it seems like we never send the maximized ones home," laughs Barb.

"I guess we have to," replies Paula. "That's all she'll allow."

Emma Stewart, seventy-three, had her right eye removed several weeks ago because of a tumor. She is mildly confused and forgetful, often angry, refusing to cooperate in the care required to heal the raw, draining wound. She shares a room with Susan Stevens, a twenty-eight-year-old woman with severe multiple sclerosis. The two spend many hours bickering, in unintelligible voices, about Emma's television, the chatter of Susan's two pet finches. Each time I pass the room I see the flickering shadows of the small black-and-white television by Emma's bed, dancing across the drawn drapes. Over the gap in her face she wears a soiled bandage. I can smell the rancid odor of illness and fear simply by walking past the door.

"Her vision's so bad she'll go into the dining room to sit down, and the chair will be three feet away," says Margery.

Nancy pushes away from the table and lifts her hands in supplication. "Well, guys, I don't know what to do with this lady. There's no way she can eat in a communal setting. She would be completely ostracized. Maybe foster care—but it would have to be a very skilled foster home to manage her."

"There's no use putting off the inevitable," says Paula. "She's never going to be pleasant to be around, and she's never going to be reliable."

Several people express the wish to see her go home, but, pressed for a reason, admit it is simply because Emma Stewart herself so wants to go home. In her confusion and misery the one thing she remembers without fail is that she wants to go home. But it is not possible: she is unsafe, unstable. She smokes without caution, falls from her chair.

"I'm not sure *we* would take her at an ICF level," says Paula. "But she *could* be managed at a lower level, so she has to go." Her wound and her troubled personality combine to make Emma Stewart *almost* "skilled"—but not quite. Harvest Moon would bump her to skilled rather than admit her to the intermediate wings, knowing how she'd benefit from the extra attention and training. But almost is not enough, and technically she doesn't qualify. As a welfare patient she has no leeway for flexible judgments, for "just this once" decisions—there are few in that bureaucracy. But Harvest Moon has no vacancies for intermediate-care welfare patients—it rarely does—and the barely functioning budget dictates that she must go, must make room for a "skilled" patient. Paula knows that the utilization review committee will kick her out at the next meeting, that further care will be denied by Medicare. Nancy must find another placement soon. Two weeks ago Paula gave Nancy two more weeks to search.

"She can't be in a situation where she would smoke unsupervised," adds Nancy, hoping for more time.

"Or *sit* unsupervised," adds Margery.

"The retirement home people would tear her apart," says Nancy in a final bid. "They'd go out of their way."

Paula, reluctantly, agrees to another week, and chalks it up as a probable denial.

Maximize, minimize. Improve, comfort, reassure. These words have little to do with the nurses on the floor and their private labors. They are code words, truncated. The nurses get to know the patients so well, with such an oddly unbalanced intimacy, that "comfort and reassurance" are bare shades of their experience. The intimacy that the nurses and aides share with their patients is born of time, embarrassment, pain, intuition, and loss, and always a kind of love; it is the kind of intimacy that families share, families whose members are so different from each other, who don't always like each other, who find themselves thrown together on the most familiar terms without recourse, and must, awkwardly, find ways to get along. Short-term goals, long-term goals: always in the mind of the nurse changing the dressing is the desire for the wound to heal, for the infection to cease and the skin to be whole again. But that desire isn't separate from skin on skin, from the exclamation of burning when the medication is applied, the tears, the pleas, the gratitude for tenderness which is no more and no less than itself—direct, exact, and real.

Nursing itself has begun to give the lie to what happens

here. It exhorts a bootstrap philosophy now, a tug of each member up to a level dictated by its most vocal leaders. The femininity of nursing, its "womanliness"—intuitive judgment, nurturing, passive acceptance of the course of events, and most of all the willingness to be the anonymous custodian of ill health's little messes—all this is discouraged, so slyly, with such forceful positiveness, by the renovation of nursing into a profession. The profession seeks to define itself, for the sake of proper compensation. A quiet word, a stroked cheek, a sharp retort held back in spite of demands and deadlines— these, too, shall be snubbed. Political leaders in the nursing profession herald a day when all nurses will have four-year-college degrees, when all nurses will be trained as administrators, teachers, researchers. They envision higher pay, more respect, more control. They see the day when nursing will be accepted as a unique profession beside medicine and law. To this end, both nationally and by state, a vocal minority of nurses is lobbying for a change in the licensure, such that to bear the coveted title "registered nurse" you must have a four-year degree.

"They can push for four-year degrees from now until hell freezes over, because they're not going to provide the ways and means to do it," says Paula, herself a two-year nurse who worked her way through a bachelor's degree program later. "When you've got a four-year degree, you've *got* to be in an administrative position, to make it worth your while to have gone to school so long. And who's going to take care of the patients?" She stabs out her cigarette and immediately lights another.

"They'll create a huge nursing shortage. And who'll suffer? The same thing that always suffers! Long-term care. The old nurses who couldn't survive twenty years ago will pull their hats out of mothballs and take a refresher course, and we'll be set back twenty years."

That dusty cap is a good example of where the idea of professionalism can go, of how cycles of image and public relations move. In the late seventies nurses began abandoning not only the starched cap, with its wings and thin black stripe, but the white leather shoes and uniforms, too, in favor of polo shirts, white jeans, and running shoes. First one hospital, then another and another gave up their strict dress codes—particularly cap requirements—as nurses protested. It is, after all, a workers' market still. I have never owned a cap—never worn one, even to look in the mirror. My own nursing school, conservative and traditional, found it impossible to keep their students' heads covered.

And suddenly in the last few years the cap is back. Dress codes are back. The cap as a symbol of nursing has returned, and in the last year Harvest Moon began requiring them again, by blanket order without room for dissent.

"I had a nurse take me aside when I first got in the industry," says Roger Scarpelli, the administrator. "She had nursed three presidents, was director of nursing at that institution, and died in that institution. She told me that the greatest honor a nurse had was her cap. And she said, 'Roger, one thing I've always admired about you is that you see to it that the nurse wears her honor on her head.' I really respect that. To me, when a person is sick, particularly the elderly and the generation we deal with—these people don't understand the new styles. They relate to the old. The cap is a symbol of security, authority. It's very relaxing. If you're lying in bed and you're blurry-eyed and you're eighty years of age, and you have someone bending over you trying to tell you, 'Take this, it's good for you'—it's just a face with no identification marks up there, it's scary. And they can't see the little pin. But if they see the white hat on the head, it's a whole different ball game. Yeah, they *will wear their hats*. It's like wearing your diploma all day long."

Janet Krause, who helped revive the dress code last year, adds, "I think the elderly look at us and say, 'Those are nurses.' It says something about us professionally and about our pride in the nursing profession. You'd be amazed at the number of comments we get from people who say, 'I like the white uniforms and I especially like the caps.' "

Janet doesn't wear a uniform or cap; she dresses in conservative dresses and a lab coat. She sees herself as separate from the floor nurses, in a different position. Paula dresses the same way, except that she isn't known for her conservatism. Today she wears pink stretch pants and a pink blouse with lavender shoes.

The nurses respond in different ways. "I was a real diehard," says Bonnie Pereira. "I waited till the last day." Erin Myers wears the cap without complaint. "It's something I take off at the end of the day. Uniforms save me shopping—I hate shopping. Besides," she adds, "patients see my cap and don't bother me for little things. They say, 'Oh, never mind, that's not your job.' It's saved me from emptying a lot of bedpans, that's for sure."

Judy Currie has decided she likes supervising, even has a talent for it, talent which takes her by surprise. "I've always had a problem with assertiveness in my life. Nurses really have a problem asking for help—they want to be super-nurse, super-mom, super-wife. We see ourselves as being the helper, not needing help." She is solemn in her task still, moving into the changed perspective of the manager so steadily she almost forgets how different the landscape looks from her new perspective.

"There are days when I've been out on the floor, helping to put a feeding tube down or giving a new medication, and the world as I knew it four months ago is very fresh in my mind again. In the few short months I've been supervising I can forget, voluntarily, what it's like out there. When you're out there there's no way to forget it." A new nurse, a fresh graduate in much the same position Judy was in a year ago, is having difficulty now. "I see her at the end of the day, in tears, falling apart. She's at the end of C Wing, the hardest assignment. She's barely managing. But she hasn't asked me for help yet." For Judy there is always another side. "Some days I think the administration really has no concept of what it's like, what they're asking us to do. But more and more I agree with them, that with changes and perseverance it can be done."

"I was in college studying animal science and got drafted," says John Eldizondo. His forearms bulge up from his shirt, thick and burly; his biceps strain the crease in his neatly ironed white shirt as he perches on the rocking patio bench in front of Harvest Moon. The barrel chest, massive shoulders, and powerful thighs are too big for his height, too big as well for the small, orderly teeth that hide in his small mouth. He wears his salt-and-pepper hair very short across the top of a large square head framed with a precise, graying beard. As he talks about his past his little gray eyes flick sideways toward me past a big Roman nose.

"I came back from Vietnam pretty screwed up and went to work in a mental institution as a nighttime aide for a year. I was planning to go to nursing school and got busted for drugs, and you can't get into nursing school when you have a felony record. It haunts me to this day.

"I got into construction work and moved out here and helped build some of the skyscrapers downtown. Then I was in a tunnel cave-in a few years back and broke my back. So I decided I'd get back into medicine again."

When John talks, he holds himself straight and full of challenge. There is in him a boy, long rejected, bred by suspicion. He expects rejection. But, for all the bone-crushing strength of his arms and all the frustration in his posture, he also holds himself with gentleness, lightly, as though he sat on his aunt's antique davenport and feared it might break. When he talks about the other aides, he calls them "frail girls," and not without affection. He calls his patients "little old ladies" with no hint of irony, without cleverness.

"If I could make it ideal, I'd make it so people had more privacy," he says. "People are supposed to *live* here. And they have no privacy. A nurse or fellow worker will come in there when I'm working on somebody, flip open the curtain, and say, 'Hi! The Celtics score is seventy-eight to sixty-seven!' That's so commonplace that I don't drop my mouth open any more when it happens. There's a nurse that won't even cover people back up when she gives an injection. But I won't name names." He grunts. "I know if I was a naked lady lying there I wouldn't feel good about it. I'm really a bug on this privacy thing.

"A lot of the older women have never been taken care of by a man before. It's really funny—men all their lives are having nurses fiddle with them and stuff like that, and now this kind of thing is flopping back on the women, with men taking care of them. I think if you handle yourself in a professional manner and don't go in there like some heathen, everything will be fine."

John has worked at Harvest Moon for a year and makes $4.40 an hour. Like many of the aides, he feels he's been overlooked for wage increases, and that almost everyone else makes more money for less work.

"It would be nice to have a six-dollar-an-hour job. Six dollars an hour would make a lot of people happier. But if you were into making money you wouldn't be in this business."

Howie Kramer is one of John's favorite people, though he thinks, like many people, that Howie's personality is changing. John's ability to lift and turn Howie without a struggle, without resorting to the hated Hoyer lift, is a gift to Howie.

"It just amazes me how some of these people can have the spirits they have. If I put myself in Howie's spot, I'd just be looking for ways to end my life."

John owns a small house a few miles from Harvest Moon. He calls it his "ball-and-chain," part of the reason he doesn't move on to something else. "Sometimes I wish I was a little freer," he says. "A job like this, you can go down and work on the coast for six months and walk in the sand every morning. You can go down to Arizona and work every winter with a job like this." A door inside the building slams, and he looks at his watch. The shift is beginning. Wistfully, he adds, "I'm kind of a chicken in that respect."

"Some are kind, some are cruel." "They kick me, I kick them." There is in the relation between patient and nurse—between sick and well, weak and strong—a kind of reciprocal poetry. The person on his back, the beetle Gerry Kennett has become against her will, cares little in the end for certification and license, niceties of distinction. Perhaps in healthier days—perhaps. But in illness we care about strength, and kindness, and the impersonal love that allows a young person on two strong legs to hold the basin while an old man throws up, and hold it gently—delicately—as though it is life itself, eggshell-thin, that is held.

"You figure if God didn't intend, you know, for *somebody* to do this kind of work, he wouldn't have given that kind of concern to people," says MaryAnn Bigler, the nurse's aide. She is unconcerned with poetry. "Me, I don't believe in religion itself, because there's too many religions. For me, it's the relationship. That's Christianity. Sometimes they need a little helping hand to give them a little more faith, help them hold on, you know, when they know they're gonna die. I think it's important to have a good Christian concern for people. It makes it a little more able to let some things slide, the way some people act, you have to let it go, you know, forgive and forget, you know, because people can't help the way they are."

At one end of D Wing, across from Cecil Lunt's room, is Grandma. Her name is Estelle Santo, but for years everyone has called her Grandma. She has never failed, in the four years I've known her, to answer the same questions exactly the same way.

"Grandma, hello, how are you?" I ask, smiling widely, for that helps.

109

"Have you ever had a birthday?" For a moment I'm confused, and then I realize the voice comes from the woman in the bed beside Grandma. She is turned away from us; I can't see her face.

"Oh, not very good, dear."

"*I* had a birthday," comes the other voice, melting into Grandma's with precision.

"Don't you feel well?" I ask, and look to the other bed, and sure enough, the moment I finish the woman there begins. "I'm ninety-one years old," she says. "How's Alan?" Grandma doesn't seem to notice.

"No, I've been sick, dear." After this rote exchange she peers at me a little closer. "Who are you, dear?" And this, too, she asks me every time.

Grandma has gained weight, putting softness in the bony face framed by an extraordinarily severe bun. Her voice drones, a monotone, edged with pique. Later in the conversation I tell her I'd come to see her a few times, but she'd been asleep.

"Well, you should pull my nose, then," she answers, a little irritated.

"You'd bite my fingers off."

"Well, I probably would, dear. So what?"

So what, indeed. Worse things happen. Erin Myers has been a nurse on the evening shift for five years, since her graduation from nursing school. She and John Eldizondo are good friends, peers in their discontent. Erin is plain of face and wears her brown hair shoulder-length and loose. She has a gruffness in her manner, a challenge, and keeps to herself. Privately she admits her unhappiness with her work, hoping to explain the feelings that seem, at first, so cold.

"The rewards are very few," she says quietly. "If I had to do it over again I'd have never gone into nursing. I can't tell you how demanding and tiring the whole thing is. All these peo-

110

ple clamoring after you, more work than you can possibly get done in a given span of time—it's almost overwhelming. I think the public image of what a nurse should be is so—it's difficult to live up to that, and it's not realistic, because you don't feel sweet and caring and giving. After a while you feel too much is being asked of you, like a person who's being pulled by all their limbs. Everybody's got a grip on you."

Erin bucked the tide last year when, after two years as the evening-shift supervisor and on the verge of a promotion to day-shift supervisor, she asked for a demotion back to the floor.

"I *hated* it," she says. "The higher up you go, the more entrenched in red tape you are, and the more you're expected to be a yes person for the administration. I can't do it. I knew that the key to maintaining sanity was to climb back down the ladder and not get so involved with initials and letters behind my name, because I'd learned by then it wasn't important to me at all."

CHAPTER NINE

Hail Fellow, Well Met

There have been no deaths for ten days, no emergencies. But the quiet is limited to that arena; it is two days till Christmas, and every year Christmas comes bearing the gifts of singing Girl Scouts, decorations, potlucks, newly inspired volunteers, visitors rarely seen, and stress.

The ceilings are strung with golden and white snowflakes. The nurses' desk is wrapped in gift wrap and ribbon. The dining room windows have been painted in scenes of snowmen and Garfield the cat dressed as Santa Claus. Almost every day another group of children—from schools, Scout troops, churches—files through the halls, singing carols in high, feathery voices and darting sidelong glances at the silent watchers in the doorways, who sit with their hands in their laps, shawls draped over their legs, heads nodding, nodding to the beat of the feet on the tile. Between the ringing of the phones a whistled "Winter Wonderland" rises and falls.

A nurse's aide coasts toward Robert Zittle, where he waits for a relative to collect him for a family feast. She is slim and slow, and walks up behind Robert in his maroon-colored polyester suit as languidly as a model on a walkway. Her skin is a

112

perfect chocolate, her makeup a perfect and exquisite rainbow. Her tiny face is framed by an Afro almost a foot wide. She slides up behind Robert and leans over his chair, places a small hand on his arm, and says, "They're here, Robert. I'll send you down to the door." And smiles. And Robert Zittle smiles back crookedly, leans on the control for his chair, and hums electrically past her to his holiday meal.

In spite of a kidney infection that sent him back to the hospital for several days, the slow, implacable Custer Holland is making dramatic progress in physical therapy. He has repeatedly surprised Martin King, who admits he ought to be immune to surprises by now. But Tillie Mott, muffled and cold and so vulnerable as to think she is naked, has made almost no progress at all. "She's a *very* hard worker," says Martin. She is confused, slow to respond, depressed. He finds it hard to justify her Medicare now, because she shows no real hope of improvement; next week she will be transferred to the ICF wing.

Verna Livingston was moved suddenly, by her family, to a small nursing home near their home. She left without a fuss, after three years at Harvest Moon. "I probably won't like it there any more than here," she carped on her last day, fingering her pearls.

Emma Stewart is gone too, to a private foster home run by a nurse. Before she left this morning she threw a glass of juice at Bonnie Pereira.

"If Emma can't make it in this home she won't make it in foster care," says Nancy Rice, with doubt in her voice. Emma packed her bags two days ago in anticipation of the move. It is her last hope, her last chance, before a permanent placement in an ICF nursing home—if any will take her.

An elderly couple stand at the desk talking to Judy Currie. The woman carries a big box of homemade fudge wrapped with a red satin ribbon. "This is for everybody who helps take care of Millie Peterson," the woman tells Judy. Millie is sitting several yards away, strapped into a wheelchair. She wears a pink jogging suit and matching running shoes. Her thin brown hair is tied back in a tight bun. She is asleep, perhaps, or simply dreaming, curled up on herself and silent. Millie hasn't spoken—or seemed to know her surroundings—in over five years, but she can move from bed to chair, feed herself with her hands, call in a strained yell when she feels uncomfortable. The woman glances at Millie and back at Judy. "We can't give *her* anything, you know, because she doesn't care. And thank you."

Roger Scarpelli is riding high: the state health department just finished their annual survey of Harvest Moon, and as they left, they complimented Scarpelli on the quality of care. The surveyors, in fact, could find only five "deficiencies," or violations, and all were minor, matters of paperwork, trivial failures to document—one was Roger's neglect to have everyone sign the roster at a lecture on fire drills. Roger feels as though he's been personally patted on the back.

"I had a family come in the other day, late in the day, and ask if they could take a look around. I said, 'Well, all my staff is gone, but I'd be glad to take you around myself.' They walked to the front door and stopped, and the woman said, 'This is where I want my brother. It smells so nice and clean.' She said they'd just been in a nursing home, and walked in, turned around, and walked out again, it smelled so bad." He smiles.

"I said, 'Well, it's not fair to judge it here. We're a long way from the problem areas. I gotta be up front with you,' I said. 'It's possible that we're gonna smell an odor because someone could have an accident. We got a lot of people here, and a lot of times the only way the nursing staff is going to become aware of a problem is by the odor.'

"I took them through and introduced them to the nursing staff and didn't talk to them after that. And they transferred the brother in two days later. Not a week goes by that I don't get a written statement from someone out there, that we have cared for a family member and they're saying thank you, and we appreciate it, and please use this donation for whatever you want. And this time the state saw that, too."

But all is not well. In the last few weeks a thief has been at work. Buddy Mullin's Sony Walkman, Susan Stevens's cassette tapes, a clock, slippers, money, and even unopened Christmas presents have disappeared. Just before the lunch hour Roger closes the door to his office and walks to the nurses' station, a grim expression on his face. He asks Judy Currie to page all the nursing staff immediately. They gather in a crowd in a few short minutes, milling quietly, a few faces worried. One nurse leans over to Addie, the therapy aide, and says, "You'd better go. You're not allowed to hear us criticized."

He briefly outlines the problem. He is emotional and gruff, looking each person in the eye in turn. Janet Krause stands nearby, nodding. He asks that people be aware of "new faces" and not hesitate to ask visitors if they need assistance.

"I will defend each and every one of my employees until proven otherwise," he says. "I will go on the premise that it is an outsider. But it may be one of our peers. Believe me, as soon as I find out, that person is gone, that day—hook, line, and sinker.

"It is worse than stealing candy from a baby, because the baby hasn't had a chance to taste the candy yet. These people have had a chance to taste life. What they have is very dear and precious to them, for whatever reason, and to rip that off them is more than stealing a radio or a clock—it's stealing life off them. I don't care if I'm in a meeting with the board, if you have an uncomfortable situation you come and get me." He shakes his head. "I know. I lose my cool. I hate this. It reflects on all of us, it reflects on the facility." He pauses. "That's all. Thank you."

Later Roger tells me about his attempt to visit a large urban nursing home in the southeastern United States. He was met at the door by a security guard who demanded his reason for visiting and then informed Roger that only immediate family, and one other person for each patient if the family allowed it, was permitted to enter. "I said. 'You've got to be kidding! You can't stop people!' And he said, 'We can and we do. Someday you'll have to do this, too.' "

Roger knows he's right. "Someday we'll have a locked door and a little camera watching you, and somebody asking through the door why you're here."

Howie Kramer signed a contract a few days ago, good for two weeks. It is signed by Janet Krause and Nancy Rice, and Howie's shaky X. In the contract—a copy of which is taped to the wall above his head—he agrees to get out of bed six days a week, using the Hoyer lift; to be turned every two hours; to be bathed on a schedule. In turn Harvest Moon agrees to teach the aides proper use of the lift, to position him comfortably; to always use two people to move him.

He is happy to see me—happy every time. He strains to remember my name, guessing wildly. Howie has decided I am his friend, and begins each conversation with comments on my hairstyle, makeup, and dress. He nearsightedly peers at my clothes and tries to guess their colors, and as soon as I smile and respond, he starts to talk, zigzagging from idea to idea along the circuitous, self-referent course.

My red sweater reminds him: "My uncle got hit by a truck because he was color-blind and walked when the light was red," Howie tells me, almost gleefully. "That was the end of him. He was just a bunch of pieces after that."

Today Howie denies the validity of the contract. He is eating a bologna sandwich, chewing while he talks, with small crumbs of crust falling onto the sheet pulled up against his chin.

"They forced me," he mumbled through a mouthful of bread. "They changed the original so I wouldn't know. They're too smart for me. My head and my feet and my stomach ache because they just leave me here, so what am I gonna do? My Christmas is already ruined." He chews a minute. "I don't want them to use the Hoyer lift. I hate it. They think I'm making a stink but I'm so contracted I keep spasming all the time." He says all this in stepped-down, sluggish rhythms. His voice begins to whine like a fan belt pulled too tightly, running against friction. "Oh, maybe not, I don't know. I feel like I'm all alone."

A young man, a nurse's aide, comes into Howie's room.

"Whatta you want?" Howie asks him, still upset.

"I just wanted to see if you'd like to visit," he answers, a little surprised at the tone. Howie shakes his head.

"No. You'd better leave. You'd get in trouble." The aide shrugs and goes. "See, that's why he left so fast. He's not supposed to talk to me. The nice aides are afraid they'll get in trouble too."

As he talks he continues to chew the sandwich, dropping whole pieces of bologna on his chest, then squinting over his body to search for them. He smells sour and wet; his face shines.

"I'm afraid of Janet, too," he adds suddenly. "Or whatever her name is. 'Cause I started to believe her and she gave me some rotten oranges and she said, 'You'd better eat them and not spit them out.' She said if I get fat she'd put me in the hospital, just because I ate two pieces of fudge! I won't get fat, I *won't!*" When I suggest that Janet wouldn't do such a thing, he gives me a pitying glance. "You just don't know."

He starts to blink suddenly and rubs his eyes with the back of his one working hand. "Oh dear, oh dear," he says. "I got mustard in my eyes." He starts to cry, a small, sad sound, as I wipe at his eyes with a wet cloth. "When I was little, little—" He is crying now, so hard he can't talk. "I know why I'm so stubborn. Because my father taught me to be-ee-ee-ee-hoo-hoo-hoo!" He sounds artificial, a little demented, like a cartoon. He raises his voice and the tears fill his eyes. "He said I wouldn't

117

get anywhere unless I waaaassss!" He hiccups a little. "Oh, if I don't quit crying I'm going to be not able to breathe!"

Later Howie has finished his sandwich, dried his eyes, and refused both the rest of his lunch and the hot-pack treatment Addie offers for his swollen right elbow. He is talking instead about Robert Zittle, who also has multiple sclerosis. For a brief time Robert and Howie shared a room.

"You know what Robert told me? If I left here I *would* die. 'Cause, other nursing homes are worse. But I don't think so. He's better than me even though he always tells me he's about to die." Howie is silent a moment, then adds, "He's eleven years older than me. I remember that."

At two in the afternoon, with the sky still chilly and brilliant, Howie is out of bed and lies tucked under a flannel sheet in a wheelchair laid almost flat. He is in the dining room with a growing crowd of people for the monthly happy hour, when beer and wine are served—to those with a doctor's permission. Today the entertainer is Jack Ryberg, who bills himself the Strumming Fool, a popular attraction at Harvest Moon. He sits on the very edge of a metal folding chair, dressed in a white shirt and black pants, with a red vest and black string tie. Jack Ryberg is about fifty years old, very tall, and friendly. He fingers the banjo in his lap a few minutes, then speaks loudly and jovially to the crowd packed haphazardly around him.

"I got a joke for you-all today," he says. "See, there was this guy from Mexico named José. And he came to the United States to visit his friend. And his friend took him to a baseball game." Jack is almost laughing already, full of the force of humor about to be unleashed. "At the start of the game everyone stood up and sang the national anthem. And then they watched the game, and afterwards José's friend asked him how he liked it. 'Well,' said José, 'you Americans are real nice. All those people wanted *me* to have the best seat.' 'Why, what do you mean,

José?' asked his friend. 'Well,' he replied, 'right there at the beginning everyone stood up and sang, 'José, can you see?' "

The Strumming Fool is pleased with himself, and doesn't seem to expect more reaction than the few isolated laughs he receives.

"Baby face!" Jack starts to sing. "You've got the cutest little baaaby face!" His voice is flat and loud, and he riffs the banjo rapidly. A few people tap the arms of their chairs and nod peacefully.

> There's not another one could *take* your place,
> *Baby* face!
> My poor *heart* is jumping—
> You sure have *started* something!

Willie, the dishwasher, is a waiter at today's happy hour. He runs madly around and between wheelchairs, balancing trays of wine glasses, blowing kisses. He pinches Phoebe White's cheek and she giggles. "Let's party!" he cries, spinning in a circle, and is gone to the kitchen for more.

There is so much white hair and paisley in this group that from my position in the back of the room I have trouble telling one person from another. The bodies are so still and slow that Willie's simple exuberance appears almost manic. His energy is like an unloosed natural force, like rapidly heating molecules of water or balloons with the air released, flying backward. The audience is vague and torpid, fatigued; their bodies, at least, grown enervated with time. It is hard, sometimes, to see what happens in the hidden places, to imagine exuberance locked inside a body whose exuberance is spent. I feel alien today, from another realm. And so I am.

Some of us are born old, and some of us grow young. If we are lucky time leaves us polished and smooth, like a sea cliff, precipitous and unobscured. But of course we never expect change at all—change always surprises, even when we long for it. It is our common arrogance to experience each small movement, each little lesson of the years as the last one, the best one from which we have no need to move again.

There is a large high school less than a block from my house, and a considerable amount of teenage foot traffic passes my way every school day. I watch them, the way they stand, the way they place themselves in relation to each other, and the way those spatial relationships change, how the young unblemished girls stroke their hair, the boys their jeans, in narcissistic concern. They move with raw and unappreciated power, the power of health and youth, sleek cats full of spring. I feel, watching them—and seeing them occasionally glance up from their labors long enough to notice me, not quite old enough to be their mother, but old, old, and then glance away, forgetting me—that I am somehow fundamentally different from them and that the difference is the product of time: that simple, that immense. The ordinary and inexorable passage of years is a force of evolution not only to the race, but to each of us on our lonely journeys. It is like the larva and the pupa that pass one into the other, and then into something else again; utterly dissimilar yet utterly the same. *Alien,* I think, is the wrong word, for there isn't in this any sense of repulsion. It is more a fascination, almost anthropological in scope. The youths pass me, I pass them, hauling children along like any adult, and smile to myself, always a little surprised, a little wistful. Everything has happened so quickly. How very different I have become from what I was! And then I look at the toddler beside me and see how very different she is in turn. Motivation and voice, language and purpose, even the quality of our skin—all different. I recognize the similarity, the racial bond, but I also see the difference.

I am occasionally asked for anecdotes, little stories to tell of the nursing home, the elderly—to explain, somehow, my presence there. I always find it hard to remember any but the most apocryphal, and those don't do justice to the daily hue and cry.

What I remember is the miniature nature of great events: small, silent moments, small snippets of conversation, small smiles of acknowledgment—and tears of bewilderment. They can't be explained and they can't be conveyed. There are stories, true, I am telling some here; but the real story has no beginning and end, no middle. It is only where I find myself in it, and by finding myself in it I can't describe it. Such a thing can't be contained, packaged, sold. I can choose to swim in the stream, or not. I can't be halfway there.

So here in this dining room, the air stirred as lazily by the fans as the bodies are stirred by the music, are roles, many roles, and many lines of separation. For a moment I stop feeling myself struck bare by time's passing. Look at all these lovely faces! Look at this exquisite prize, this humanness in all its forms. I cherish the difference, and the sameness, and for a moment find that *I* am passing through time, which stands patient and still, and waits for me to catch up. It is like a rumbling in the earth, a rolling thunder, a tattoo of drums pounding deep and distant, a vibration in the ground beneath my feet—the force of time passing, a turning of the great and ponderous wheel, rocking my world, paying no heed. In this room are my past and present and future, myself with yesterday's ignorance and tomorrow's spent exuberance, and me. The separation blurs; we are all engaged in a most absorbing experiment in connectedness. It is the elimination of alienness, a scene absurd and touching. I am already old, and it is fine.

A wine glass falls and shatters, and Willie prances by with a broom, undisturbed. Cathy Bosley brings Howie a Coke and holds it gently out to him, the straw bent, so he can sip, while the Strumming Fool sings.

> Make my bed and light the light,
> I'll be home, late tonight.
> Blackbird, bye bye.

CHAPTER TEN

Gainful Employment

Over Christmas the snows came again. Soon it will be the New Year. Addie, the physical therapy aide, is poking her finger at Gina Tyrell, a nurse's aide who has worked on B and D wings for several years, berating her for living just a mile or two away.

"You can *walk* home from here," says Addie.

Gina looks at her stonily. "Your *mama.*"

Addie walks away, mumbling. "I'm going to the hospital and checking myself in," she says.

Paula Schulz is sorting through piles of paper on her desk, starting to compile her yearly statistics. "One of my *favorite* jobs," she says. She is wearing a purple and pink flowered blouse, with neon lilac stretch pants and a matching vest. She has several small gold chains around her neck and pink pearls stuck in her earlobes. The phone rings and she answers in a loud, jovial voice.

"What's happening?" She listens and stops smiling. Her voice drops. "Oh, that's too bad, Dutch." Dutch is a resident at the retirement center associated with Harvest Moon; Paula has helped him with minor illnesses in the past. "A lump in your throat? Oh, dear." Her voice is honey-soft now, her face smooth with concern. "I'll come see you after lunch. And don't you worry." She hangs up the phone gently.

Admissions drop a little over the Christmas holidays every year, because doctors try to avoid elective surgeries like hip replacements then. But winter always adds its own share of falls and heart attacks and great stone weights of depression, and the drop is usually a short one. Soon enough people are knocking on the door, calling, asking for a room, for help.

Rhonda Purcell is often the first person families meet when they inquire about Harvest Moon. She is responsible for questions, tours, helping people sort out their Medicare coverage. She must juggle ratios of money and medical diagnoses, numbers of feeding tubes in relation to bedridden patients in relation to empty beds in relation to how many welfare clients the facility is carrying. She must know how many of which kind of bed are available, or soon to be available, throughout the facility: some beds are strictly for Medicare, others strictly private. Some beds can "swing," or be used for different payment schemes as necessary. A lot of the moves within the facility—such as from one end of B Wing to the other—are because of the bed designation. Rhonda has to know not only that there are four vacancies, but that, say, two are Medicare only, three are male only, one is welfare and female and intermediate care only—and still compare it to the patient population and the nursing load at the time. It is her job to say no as often as yes. She used to ask people for financial information on the telephone, but found herself buried by sad stories and pleas for assistance.

"I tell people the rate. If they can't afford it, they can't move in," she says now. "My job's really simple. Maybe one out of twenty that I turn away bothers me, but it's because they look at me in a certain way or remind me of my mother. All personal stuff like that."

Rhonda is from the hill country of Kentucky, a big woman with large round breasts that lead her when she walks. She tapers to a remarkably thin waist, to long slim legs and tiny feet. Rhonda enjoys seeing how her clothes affect a person's response to her; she dresses one day in a tight fluffy sweater and tight jeans, another in an impeccable black wool suit. Long, thin brown hair hangs beside her round face like draperies separated by her large glasses. Rhonda smiles a lot, when she says no as well as when she says yes. She is pragmatic to a fault, free of dissembling or apology. Her own "sentimental mistakes" amuse her.

"This one guy came in for his wife, and she had a feeding tube. We weren't going to take any more since we were up to fourteen or fifteen, which is a lot for the nurses. He wasn't looking for sympathy. Just said that he and his wife were moving to a new apartment from the home they'd lived in, and she had a stroke, and if she was here he could still come and see her 'cause the new apartment was nearby." Rhonda smiles now as she talks in a deceptively diplomatic Southern twang, soft and sweet. "What could I say? I admitted her. I called Janet and said, 'We *have* to take her.' "

If a potential patient can afford the care one way or the other Rhonda starts looking for other problems. She considers whether it is, as Nancy Rice might say, a "hopeless case," likely to fill a bed for a long time—which, though economically sound, isn't compatible with the rehabilitation efforts Harvest Moon is known for. She looks at how difficult the nursing care will be: wounds, tubes, breathing problems—and weight. These patients are much more difficult to care for. "I tell my fat aunt she'd better watch it, 'cause we wouldn't take her." Rhonda tries to avoid admitting young patients, preferring to focus on the elderly; she also discourages very tall men—only three beds are over six feet long.

One of her most difficult, and common, problems is the confused patient, especially, she adds, the ones who "look normal." But now and then Rhonda looks for just such a person. "Take Millie Peterson's room. Now, that's a hard room to fill. We've got a food thrower in there. It was worse when she was a screamer, too. I have to place another confused patient to fill the other bed. A lot of it is timing. Someone might get in as a welfare patient or a terminal patient this week and not next week."

After work Rhonda and her husband ride with their friends in a motorcycle club, to bars and parties. She calls herself rowdy, and then adds, "But I get along fine with normal people." She began as a part-time clerk in the tiny medical records department six years ago, and little by little learned the intricate administrative details of Harvest Moon. When the increased turnover made an admissions coordinator a necessity, Rhonda was the obvious choice.

Much of her time is spent on the telephone with hospital social workers who are trying to place patients on short notice. "They don't exactly tell the truth," she says. "You ask them, 'Is this person a screamer?' And they say, '*Noooo!*' And if they went and looked at the charts they'd know he screamed all night." Another "misinterpretation of the facts" involves Medicaid, or welfare. A social worker might suspect that a patient is planning to apply for welfare and not tell Rhonda that little bit of information. Rhonda admits the person as a private-pay patient, only to find that their funds are about to run out. Harvest Moon has one more welfare patient than planned, and the budget has to find a place for him. "I haven't called anyone a liar yet," she adds. But the truth is not always a pragmatic choice, and Rhonda knows this, too. She knows precisely why the hospital social workers fail to tell the whole story, because it is partly her job to find placements for patients who no longer can be accommodated at Harvest Moon. "You have to lie sometimes in this job," she says. "Some people would never be placed if you told the truth about them."

Cecil Lunt, whose behavior caused serious problems for

years, Howie Kramer, Buddy Mullin, and many other patients don't fit—may have never fit—the desired model. All were originally expected to stay short times, receive therapy, and be transferred elsewhere. All are now long-term welfare residents. "We're not going to kick them out on the street," says Rhonda. "Cecil's been here for years, and we'd never ask him to leave no matter what he did. Especially since the family paid their money all that time. I guess we think he has a right to be here now."

At Harvest Moon memos circulate continually, as though with lives of their own. It is difficult to throw anything away; it is easy to imagine oneself sweating in the witness box, wishing in vain for a piece of paper discarded years before. Each day Rhonda Purcell types a memo listing the day's admissions and discharges, birthdays, the current census, changes in patients' financial information, addresses, even which funeral home a person has chosen. If anything changes—and it often does—she'll type another, canceling an admission, adding another. The memos go to Roger and Janet, to Paula Schulz and Judy Currie, to Bonnie Pereira and the other nurses on the floor, to Janet's assistant, and to Edie Douglas, Roger's administrative assistant; the memos are given to the medical records coordinator, the billing office, all the therapists, visiting hospital social workers, and home health nurses. Lab work is requested and filed in triplicate. Physician's orders are written in one, two, five different places.

All the paper exists not only to communicate, but to justify—in case of future lawsuits, in case of trouble with payment. For all the enormity of Medicare in terms of paperwork, interpretation, and effort, it pays less than five percent of the $30 billion spent annually in this country on nursing home care. And remember, private insurance pays another very small fraction, because very few insurance plans pay for more than a few weeks of skilled nursing care, and almost never any of the costs of intermediate care. It is a piece of fine print often forgotten by people when they buy insurance, preoccupied as they are with visions of huge emergency room and intensive care bills. Well and good to have those bills covered—but the aftermath of an emergency is often a long convalescence, and sometimes a permanent one.

Almost half of those billions are paid by individuals and their families. A bed in Harvest Moon's intermediate-care wing, in a room shared by three people who share their bathroom in turn with three *more* people, costs about $55 a day. Meals and nursing care are included, but not medication, doctor's visits, therapy, or supplies. In the skilled wing the cost is closer to $80 a day, and can go up, depending on the patient's needs. (Remember, too, that after the twenty-first day in a skilled nursing home, Medicare pays for all *but* the first $50 a day.) Such costs destroy a family's financial security very quickly, and there is usually no alternative to the welfare system. The social service establishment calls this process "impoverishment," the creation of a new class of poor—people who had never been poor before. The other half of annual nursing home costs, but for those small fractions, is paid by Medicaid, the federal medical care program for the poor. It is a mutually antagonistic relationship, that of the nursing home and the welfare system; one wants, the other one has; one gives, the other takes. Which is which is open to debate.

Medicaid is supposed to pay about seventy percent of the true cost of care. In 1979—statistics are slow in coming—Medicaid sponsored almost 600,000 people in skilled facilities and almost 800,000 in intermediate-care facilities. About eighty-three percent of them were over sixty-five.

Harvest Moon is paid about $42 a day for each welfare patient, whether it is Howie Kramer or Millie Peterson or Phoebe White. The rate can change, a little at a time, depending on the amount of deficit and fat in the state budget. It seems easy enough to cut the rate by a dollar a day, as recently happened in this state, and it adds up to a tidy savings for a state that supports thousands of poor people in nursing homes for years at a time. But the nursing home is under constant pressure to increase its staffing ratios, to raise salaries, improve the facility, buy air conditioning, sprinkler systems, new equipment—and pay off the old loans on the property and the building. Lawns, parking lots, dishwashers, furnaces, and telephone systems must all be kept up. The true cost for each intermediate-care patient is closer to $60 a day, and any cut seems to be too much.

To qualify for welfare you have to be poor. In many cases this means selling your home and using almost all of your savings. A lot of people try to circumvent this problem by "spending down" their assets before they get sick, or selling their house to their children for a few dollars. But to be eligible for welfare you can't do this within two years of applying. Intent counts here; if a woman has sold her home and cashed in her stocks in order to pay the medical bills for her husband, and then needs medical care herself, she would probably be accepted in spite of the "spend-down." But middle-class people, especially in retirement, will lose their assets fast enough when illness strikes without warning, as it struck Conrad Berry, in his apparent vigor, and laid him suddenly on his back at $20,000 a year. The Congressional Budget Office released figures in the late seventies indicating that almost half of all welfare patients in nursing homes had not been poor before their illness, but were impoverished by their care.

A lot of nursing homes simply won't take patients on welfare—some even advertise this fact, thinking to entice people with a class bias. In Seattle, not long ago, a 102-year-old woman who was almost completely helpless after several strokes was evicted from the home where she'd lived for eight years. She had outlived her trust fund, and had no more resources; the home where she lived didn't accept welfare patients.

The nursing home industry historically complains about overregulation by state and federal governments. But one place where there is little effective regulation—not surprisingly, considering that nursing homes are considered businesses like any other—is in profit margins. Some states limit the amount of reimbursement a home can receive but not its rate of profit, thereby holding down income without holding down the amount of money that owners can claim as their own. It is an invitation to the poorest of care, all corners cut, all expenses spared. Only the willingness of the owners to forgo potential profits is in the way.

One western state has reimbursed some profit-based nursing homes for staff travel to conventions in both Florida and Hawaii. The meetings were necessary, said the head of a state-wide nursing home industry lobby, "to build rapport" with the state and federal officials who also attended. The state also pays homes for depreciation of company-owned cars—in some cases, Jaguars, Cadillacs, and Rolls-Royces. When the state threatened to change the regulations to prevent such payments, nursing home owners warned that it would spell bankruptcy for a few facilities, and lead to poor care in others.

"Those of us who have suffered during the last two or three years from unreasonable ceilings established by states . . . know that there is no longer any fat to cut from the Medicaid cow." So writes the author of an article in *Nursing Homes,* a magazine for administrators of proprietary, or profit, nursing facilities. The author begins reasonably enough, outlining the problem intermediate-care facilities have with the crunch from DRG regulations, which are forcing nursing homes to put much more weight into skilled care. But his solution—solution, that is, to diminishing profit margins—begins to take on a chilling tone, the more so for being uttered in the slightly pained voice of an unjustly injured but reasonable man. "Those who can afford to take care of themselves will want quality," writes the author. "They have been used to it and it is what they will demand with their dollars. . . . We shall start to discriminate in favor of those who have the ability to pay. That certainly does not mean we shall discriminate against those who do not have the ability to pay. They will be provided with proper care, but they do not have to be provided with all the extra services at a level equal to those who have the ability to pay. . . . There will be the minimum but acceptable quality of life."

He fails to enumerate the "extra services," even though he returns to them again and again in the course of his writing, calling them by other names: "amenities," "luxury." Does this mean cable television and menu choices, or does it mean more than one aide for twenty bedridden patients? (I wouldn't be so quick, having worked in both profit and non-profit nursing homes, to assume the former.) The connection is clear that within a wide range of circumstances the quality of patient care is *directly* tied to the staff-to-patient ratio. Not sometimes, not indirectly, not statistically—it is a hard and true fact. Time, time, lack of time—labor beyond available time, lists of tasks too long for the time allotted, whispered requests and angry demands which can't be met because there is no time. Time isn't all, but it is a great deal, because it is the preciousness of time that creates the stress, the burnout, the resentment, the divisive frustration so frequently found. And staff costs are the biggest chunk of the pie, the biggest bite of the profit margin.

The author finishes with cheer: "The future is bright," he adds, for facilities willing to expand into skilled care and other services. "It is now possible to get off the sinking Medicaid ship . . . [if] you want to get a proper return on your investment and provide the best possible care. . . ." Spend-down will stop, he suspects, in favor of "advanced funding"—saving money for those golden years—because of "the realization that those who give away their assets to relatives prior to entering a nursing home simply will relegate themselves to a more basic level of care, perhaps a lower quality of life. . . ."

A friend of mine is a director of nursing at a suburban nursing home. She has garnered a reputation for solving problems. Several months ago, before she was hired as director of nursing, this facility had lost both its Medicare and Medicaid eligibility, a drastic move reserved by the state to punish severe and usually repeated violations of standards. My friend was hired to pull it up from that depth, to dig in and solve the problems. And she's done that—the rooms are clean and sunny, the floors shiny, and the beds made. The patients are clean, well-fed, their wounds treated—it's a nice place, a place I feel comfortable in. She did this by exciting the staff into believing it could be done, and by hiring new—*more*—staff. She has, as she puts it, "several times the required amount" of staff—but the home is still losing money. In a few more months she hopes it will turn around. A bad reputation can be hard to beat; she still has vacancies to fill. But I suspect my friend isn't long for this job, because the home was bought a few weeks ago, without warning, by one of the largest nursing home corporations in the country. The administrator is quitting, refusing in advance to work for them. The corporation, still unseen, has already fired the dietician and begun to switch to its own institutional meal plan. The home will be expected to show a profit as soon as the sale is complete—and there is only one way to do it.

"There are some things about the job I really get sick of—things that should be controllable that are out of control. But things like Medicare, Medicaid, I've always viewed as a real challenge," says Paula Schulz. Part of her job involves reporting to the Utilization Review Committee, compiling those beloved statistics—also for the URC—and challenging denials. "I've always loved doing the juggling act," she adds. Juggling is one of Paula's hobbies, one of her talents, and she does it with more than one ulterior motive. She likes the idea of beating a giant bureaucracy at its own game, playing by its rules, and she also likes the small heroic gestures she can sometimes make—keeping a patient a few days longer, uncertain of payment, or finding a way to provide a particular treatment not ordinarily covered. She likes tilting at the government windmills, playing Robin Hood for the poor and old.

"We're not gonna kick them out in the street." Paula says this, Roger Scarpelli and Nancy Rice say this. It is said with a touch of pride and anger, a righteous indignation. Such stubborn determination costs Harvest Moon, and rewards it in other ways.

Susan Stevens is twenty-eight years old. She's been in Harvest Moon for almost four years, and most of that time she's been on welfare. She has multiple sclerosis and is severely disabled: unable to speak, she cries and screams in a grating combination moan and yowl, unable to swallow and so fed by a tube, unable to control her bladder and so catheterized, subject to frequent bladder infections. She has no movement in her legs and little in her arms: little sensation except pain; her vision is poor and very sensitive to light. Her emotions are short-circuited, too, like Howie Kramer's—only with a mad cat's intensity. She cries, screams, curses, struggles and fights, then withdraws to a sluggish silence. Years ago Susan signed a Living Will, and several times has asked that it be put into effect—that the tube be removed. More than once she has asked in her awkward, halting way, not to be treated with antibiotics for a bladder infection. But then she changes her mind, the tube goes back in, the antibiotics begin again. Whether Susan Stevens is even able to make competent decisions for herself is open to debate.

At one time the Medicaid liaison decided she could be moved off C Wing—where she has lived amidst the skilled patients because of her tube, cared for by registered nurses as well as aides—and go to a cheaper bed in another, less expensive facility. But Paula and several other nurses and aides, recruiting Susan's physician, managed to convince the state that her care was so complex, her condition so mutable and unstable, that she should not be moved, that the expense should be borne. In fact, part of their argument was that it was their excellent nursing care that had kept Susan out of the hospital, kept her from repeated infections and crises—all of which would cost the state far more. It was a surprisingly sensible decision. And by

their efforts, Paula and the other nurses granted themselves unknown months and years more of caring for Susan Stevens,
who is difficult, wearing, and bound to die—who is not easy to
love, and seems at times to invite irritation. They are pleased
with the victory; like Margery Todd, Paula and her nursing
peers feel the safety—the survival—of fragile people is in their
hands. They feel it like a personal weight, and the dollar be
damned.

The work of the fiscal manager is a three-card trick, a leger-
demain of the ledger. Month by month, Harvest Moon slips
from the black to the red to the black, the play sometimes only
a thousand dollars out of a hundred thousand. Roger feels he
can, at last, point to the specific reasons for red months—bad
weather, with charges to the taxi services for ferrying staff, or
the holidays, with fewer admissions. As long as he knows
where the problems lie, he still controls the big picture. And
Harvest Moon is decidedly non-profit. In the past this was an
excuse for continual debt, but Scarpelli sees it differently.

"Non-profit doesn't mean we're not attempting to make a
profit, but we have a different profit motive," he says. "I think
that's the key. We generate income or money to be directly recycled back in to the facility and the care. It is generated to be a
benefit to other people.

"Now, if we have a lot of Medicaid patients in this facility,
and someone's trying to give us another extremely heavy-care,
difficult Medicaid patient, we may say no. Because Medicaid is
a very costly operation for us. We do not have classified patient
care. Everyone is entitled to the same level of care. The people
out there on the floor don't know if it's a Medicaid or Medicare or private-paying patient, and it's not their job to know,"
he says. "But we in the administration *do* know what it's cost-
ing us. It costs us thirty percent of our costs every day, and
that's pretty damned expensive."

But the nurses *do* know—they know because they know the
patients well, and the patients' families. They are privy to their

worries and fears, their changing status in relation to the world at large. They know because Harvest Moon uses three different lab requisitions now, to ease its own billing system: one for Medicare, one for Medicaid, and one for private pay. They know because it is part of their job to know the needs and losses of their patients' private lives, and how their illnesses change their lives. The point is that they don't care.

Roger says he's been in a few facilities across the country that exceed the quality of care given at Harvest Moon. "But they deal strictly with very high- and middle-income people, strictly private," he points out. Harvest Moon not only has lower compensation for its labors, but more regulations to cope with by handling Medicare and Medicaid claims. "Yet you want to have the same standards. Sometimes it gets pretty rough. The state doesn't compensate a fair return for the services it expects. So we have to ask people to work at a salary that is not really at a level supportive of a family. The compensation that's being paid to nurse's aides, housekeepers, the real workers—the government is unable to recognize that as a worthy service. It should be six dollars an hour. But there's no way they're going to compensate us for six dollars an hour. We'd go broke. It's impossible."

Roger Scarpelli is paid in the range of $45,000 a year. Janet Krause and Paula Schulz make almost $30,000 a year. The lowest-paid workers at Harvest Moon are called support workers, young people who help with the smoking program and meals. They are paid minimum wage. Nurse's aides start at $4.15 an hour, practical nurses at $6.70 an hour. Registered nurses who work on the floor, like Erin Myers and Bonnie Pereira, begin at $9 an hour, only three-fourths the salary they could make in a local hospital, caring for four or five patients a shift instead of twenty. Harvest Moon, even with that one-to-twenty ratio so many staff dislike, has more nurses and aides available on every shift than required by the state. Over 130 people work in the home, to provide for less than a hundred patients.

In the therapy department the aides are paid similarly to practical nurses, but Martin King and Nancy Rice and Barb Coulter, as heads of their individual departments, make considerably more—more than floor nurses.

"The budget? Oh, well, shoot. Let's cut Mr. Scarpelli's salary," says aide Mickey Bestler. "Some of these people pay over fifteen hundred dollars a month to stay here, right? I don't even make six hundred a month. That money's going somewhere besides paying for the rent of the room. And, okay, like those little tiny powder things? For the bath? They charge these people two bucks for one of those. They charge them a dollar fifty for one razor. Shit like that. Now if they're making so goddamn much money, where is it all going? *Somebody's* pocketing it—it sure isn't going to the care. They charge them for *every*thing."

When Roger Scarpelli started his job here he designated reserved parking spaces for administrative personnel. Roger, Janet, Paula, and several others in management have parking spaces near the rear entrance. Almost half of the spaces are reserved for tenants in the neighboring retirement center, and for visitors. The parking lot is usually full by midmorning, and every day a few staff members have to park on side streets and walk around the long cyclone fence that encloses Harvest Moon. Several employees simply park in visitor and tenant spaces, habitually ignoring the rule. At the last staff meeting Roger circulated a memo, and a copy was posted on the front door.

DO NOT PARK IN TENANT SPACE, it read in bold, felt-tip ink. MOVE YOUR CAR. YOU WILL BE TOWED.

CHAPTER ELEVEN

Decline and Fall

The rains have returned, warm and mild, flooding the gutters still cluttered with autumn's leaves. In the late morning a slow and solemn crowd trails to the back parking lot, almost aimless, as though on a reluctant mission. There is Roger Scarpelli in a dark gray suit, Janet Krause and Nancy Rice and Rhonda Purcell in heels and stockings and dark winter dresses. It is exactly as it appears, a funeral procession. "I hate funerals," Roger mumbles as he walks through the drizzle to his car. On New Year's Eve two cars collided on an empty stretch of road south of the city. One was driven by Linda Schulz, Paula's twenty-two-year-old daughter. She survived two days in intensive care, with massive head injuries, and finally died.

Team conference has been rescheduled, and it is almost two before most of the group assembles for the task. Paula Schulz is absent, and it's just as well: the first two patients that Nancy Rice presents to the team, both new admissions, are grim, their injuries ironic.

Jim Taub is nineteen years old, with, as Nancy points out, a history of impulsive and destructive behavior. Recently he has been involved heavily in drugs. He has been admitted to Harvest Moon for long-term therapy to overcome, if possible, the brain damage caused by a gunshot wound to his head several weeks before. Jim Taub looks quite awful, a stubble of hair filling in where his scalp was shaved for surgery, carrot-colored and coarse, one eye swollen shut and draining, that side of his face limp and flabby. He makes his stuttering way down the hall in his wheelchair, almost limping the vehicle along with unsteady tugs of his slippered feet. His one good eye drifts sideways, full of challenge. In the few days since his admission, Jim has refused to accept limits—on smoking, sleeping, bathing—though he can barely walk and can't dress or feed himself. He says he has "unfinished business" to attend to, and wants to go.

"Watch the doors," says Charlene Parrott. "I see the typical left-hemi impulsive behavior—got things to do, gotta go. No judgment." Damage to the left half, or hemisphere, of the brain causes a different kind of defect than damage to the right half. Left-hemisphere damage, whether caused by a stroke or a wound—like a shotgun blast—is characterized by impulsiveness. The ability to recognize patterns is damaged, so that cause and effect, limits, even the person's own lost abilities, are denied. Jim Taub is, as Charlene says, typical: he cannot understand why he must stay in this place, be tied in this chair, be forced away from the door.

Bruce Leonard is on Nancy's list too. He is seventeen. Over the Christmas holiday he was in a car accident involving several people, in which he was thrown from the car and suffered a serious head injury. He can't speak but sometimes follows directions slowly. He is incontinent and only now beginning to walk again. His attention span is very short and he gets easily upset—and then he screams. Bruce's father visits his son every day, exhorting the boy through each bite he painfully lifts to his mouth, each step. His brothers and sister and grandparents come regularly.

"We want to make him the best he can be," says Charlene.

The newspapers are full of the stories. It is easy to glance at them with a distracted and pitying attention. "In critical condition," "injured and in serious condition," "critical with massive head injuries." Most of us read with distraction because we are unfamiliar with the face on the head which has been so bluntly broken, with its irreplaceable expressions—nor do we pause to imagine, as we turn the page, what such phrases mean, how lives change in the fraction of a moment, in the blur and slide of a car, a pole, a ditch. Paula Schulz knows—it's her job. Bruce Leonard is one of the better results; Buddy Mullin something less. As the staff members describe the condition, debate the treatment, in place of Bruce Leonard and Jim Taub they see Linda Schulz, who used to visit her mother at work now and then—sleeping in the curious sleep of the comatose, with all the concomitant intimacies of I.V. and airway and the deep steady breath of the ventilator. And they see her buried.

Death is so much a part of the daily routine that Bonnie Pereira, talking about a longtime patient who died a few weeks earlier, can say, "It sounds kind of callous, but I didn't take note of it. She died on my day off."

Death is, in fact, so routine that nurses develop intuitive theories to account for its odd habits. (Not such a common thing, really—about forty-five people are admitted each month, and about forty-five people are discharged—not always, of course, the same ones—and on the average only four of them die. In the last three months fifteen people have died. It is a big number to anyone unused to death. The nurses hardly pause in their steps to wonder. Death has a commonness all its own, a normality; where else is death unsurprising?) The mythos, fueled by an abundance of anecdotes, has three main parts: that death comes in triads, that sleepy, half-conscious people wake a few days before they die, and that people don't die until they are given permission.

There is even a theory called transfer trauma, with documentation to back it up, that says when people are moved from one place to another—say, from hospital to nursing home—their risk of dying increases. (Transfer trauma wasn't given a nod with the DRGs; a preliminary report prepared for Congress predicted from the beginning that, while the average length of a patient's stay in any facility would decrease, the number of transfers, admissions, and readmissions would increase.) Transfer trauma only makes manifest the issues of illness: the familiar has been stolen, the fragile body stressed, surrender demanded, a greater jeopardy granted. Dying is inconvenient and troublesome, a simple process which never proceeds apace.

"In twelve years I've done a lot of it," says MaryAnn Bigler, referring to the hours at the bedside of a person dying. "It takes a lot of guts to take care of the terminals. It's hard on the feelings 'cause you get close to them. We've had some that we just bawl like babies after they go, you know. But if you have the feeling inside that at least you've made their last minutes, the time that they *were* there, worth something, that you showed them somebody *did* care, then it's okay.

"You try to make them as comfortable as you can, tell them that you care, tell them that you love them. Then they give you a smile and thank you for caring. I've met a lot of terminals, and I like taking care of them."

MaryAnn really does "bawl like a baby." It is a dramatic sight, this heavy, short woman with her hair in curls, mascara staining her cheeks as the tears run. In spite of her ineloquent classifications, the almost crude execution of her determined sympathy, MaryAnn's hand is a gift, freely given, with a value all its own. "You don't get *used* to it, someone dying, you just learn to accept it, learn to live with it as a part of life. Then you know they're gone and they weren't like that half an hour before. And you know they wouldn't want a stranger there."

How, though, can we not be strangers at such moments? The gulf is enormous. The sense of deviation, of difference, seems so real—and not only physically. Dying and dead people do look different, but there's much more at play: they *act* differently, in the most extreme way. They are *dying,* and how could a person violate the social contract more explicitly than that? There is a danger, too, of projecting your own imagined experience onto another's, of facing, when you face the dying, the terrors of one's own inevitable turn. To become not a stranger at the moment when one person is utterly, completely, finally leaving without a backward glance requires not intimacy, but distance. Oddly enough, you have to back up, step away. You have to escape the seductive preoccupation that beckons, and at the same time the desire to turn and run, to scorn.

I have seen people die since my first days as an aide. One of the oddities of the nursing home is that one is so frequently elsewhere, so often traveling between destinations. Whether it is a need for privacy, my own failure to read the subtle clues of a foregone conclusion, or some unnamed physical wisdom, I don't know—but like most nurses I am often out of the room for the moment of death. The moment, that is, of the last breath, the stilling, the sudden, delicate settling of cells. I am there, and then gone for linen or a cloth—and in that time my patient has bid farewell.

In a sense all of long-term nursing is a death watch, which bothers me not at all, because I think all of life is a death watch. But certain deaths I remember, because of how they surrounded me, of how I was enveloped for a time in their colossal, world-shaking motion. I remember one death, and a death watch, from one of my first shifts as a supervisor, alone on a weekend, tentatively in charge of the aides, the patients, the other nurses. I walked carefully and tensely through the halls. One of my many charges that day was Pearl, who had been declining for months. She was an obese and silent woman, fed by a tube and the slow spoonfuls of puree offered by the aides. She watched the proceedings around her with what appeared to be a jaded and critical eye. She never spoke, or cooperated, but neither did she fight. She simply allowed, without protest, the care we gave. She had a mild case of pneumonia, which we treated, by the family's wish, without great effort, and sooner or later she was bound to die from it.

Pearl's aide that morning was a young, frizzy-haired girl named Liz, new to the nursing home, as tentative as I. She watched Pearl's stertorous breathing with rapt and fearful attention. Several times in the morning Liz asked me to come look at Pearl, listen with what she assumed were more experienced ears. Finally I called the priest listed on Pearl's chart, and tried, without success, to call a relative. The priest came, jovial and kind, and pulled up a chair to Pearl's bed to read his Bible. He murmured to her, turning the pages. She watched him, the wall, the movements of the nurses, with equally distant interest. At last the priest carefully adjusted his vestments and read the Last Rites, forming a solemn slow cross above her still body. She watched.

About twenty minutes after he left, Liz found me, tearful. "I don't think Pearl's breathing," she whispered. I realize now, though it didn't occur to me then, that Liz somehow thought she was responsible for Pearl's death. "I was feeding her and she just—stopped."

And Pearl was dead, and dead she was different—what was still and distant before was a complete absence now. She was sitting up in bed, propped with pillows to be fed, her head lolling on her neck. Her skin was already waxen, and I imagined I could feel it begin to cool under my hand. It was as though the hairs on her arms themselves had died. In my own tense inexperience I began the rote tasks, the list of protocol to follow. I'm still sorry I didn't take a few moments to explain them to Liz, to take *her* by the hand. I sent her for wet warm washcloths and towels, lowered the bed so that Pearl lay flat. I pulled out the feeding tube and threw it away, cut off and removed the catheter that had drained her urine. Liz returned and together, behind the curtains, we gave Pearl a bath, dressed her in a clean gown, and pulled the sheet up to her chest. Liz did as I asked, quiet and shaky. She looked at me, a little startled, when I whispered to Pearl, telling her what we were doing.

And then I called the funeral home, and finally reached one of her daughters, and explained. The men in dark suits with the long black bag came and rolled Pearl away. I went back to my medicine. Two weeks later Liz quit.

The fabric of acceptance, the tempered tolerance of natural death, is torn by the unnatural ones—the deaths we try to prevent. This is the going on and on of Conrad Berry and his kin, the suspension in tubes and dreams of lives saved, pulled back from the precipice. And there is a terrible march of predictability to such a death, a sameness that is almost a parody. Having seen it many times before, I can look at Irma Washington, Conrad Berry, even Cecil Lunt, and tell you not only what they will die from, but how they will get to that peaceful place.

This is only one way—there are many, of course, many escapes for people like Cecil and Conrad—heart and lungs, kidney and liver and pancreas. And this one is not so bad, not as bad as it sounds. (There are worse, chilly winds all—and who knows the experience, the knowledge of it? The survivors, those few whose hearts stopped, whose breathing failed, who claim they flew out of their body to a kind of heaven and then returned—the survivors call it grace. They say the manner of death is of little importance, once it's done.) But this is one way: I've seen it many times. The feeding tube will become dislodged—pulled out by a desperate or uncomprehending hand, tugged accidentally by a sheet or gown. It may take weeks or months, but eventually the tube will slip from the stomach— just an inch or two—and before the nurse finds it, formula will drip, a few secretions perhaps, into the lungs. From this grows aspiration pneumonia.

Even without a tube, without a single mortal mistake, pneumonia can come. It is called "the old man's friend," the disease of the bedridden, of lungs flattened under weight and age and motionlessness. And with pneumonia comes viscid, copious mucus in the lungs and throat, which must be suctioned out—at first a few times a day, then many times, then hourly and more—by delicate, translucent vacuum tubes that suck out oxygen as well, so that every few seconds the nurse will pause and wait for a little color to return to the suddenly gray cheeks, the distress to leave the sleepy face. Because of the pneumonia and the secretions and the suctioning, oxygen cannula—little plugs that fit in the nose, and dry out the membranes till they crack and bleed—are added, for the comfort of easily breathed air. The pneumonia brings fever, and fever is bad for the skin, especially skin that lies most of the time in bed. Since the person is comatose, or nearly so, the urine and feces pour unnoticed into the bed. (Most comatose people have Foley catheters inserted permanently into the bladder to drain off urine. Sooner or later catheters and incontinence lead to bladder infections.) It is in this soup that bedsores are born, in spite of vigilance and exhaustive effort. Sweat, oil, urine, feces, and weight, friction, and pressure demand a toll—and remember, I am talking not about a few days, but of weeks and even months. Aspiration pneumonia is not a fast and lethal illness. It lingers.

There are wonderful beds, specially made of odd mixtures of sand or water or air bubbles or beads, that slide and vibrate and roll under a bedridden person, massaging and soothing the skin, wicking away moisture, softening the blow of rolling over. These are fascinating things, these beds, taking on the unique shape of whoever lies in them, molding themselves to the bones. They cost not a few thousand dollars, but many tens of thousands of dollars. Large hospitals may have—on lease—a few. Nursing homes haven't any. Foam mattresses and alternating air-pressure mattresses and soft, furry white sheepskin pads are the only helpmates for the two or three people who come every few hours—who have twenty people, remember, to come to as often as possible, turning, massaging, molding the world as best they can. And sooner or later the skin on the hips, the heels, the elbows, the shoulder blades turns red and mushy, spills open, drains its own contribution to the soup. The fever pitches and rages, and perhaps this person, receiving—of course—the best of attention, is on antibiotics, battling the pneumonia, hanging on.

The stroke patient who dies after months in a coma is the result of a few days of highly skilled labor by a specially trained hospital staff, who manage, with the best of intentions, to keep this stranger from the streets alive. And when the extent of the loss is understood—when it becomes obvious that the person has no "potential for rehabilitation"—he or she is transferred to a nursing home. No one calls it a mistake, questions the correctness of the effort made. But the nurses and the aides who embrace the result share a fundamental difference in desire from the physicians and nurses who create it. They care for people who have become no longer strangers, and this is a powerful thing to become. They have become real.

Cardiopulmonary resuscitation (CPR) is the standard practice when a person's heart stops or they stop breathing. It is supplemented by a rush and flurry to the hospital, where chemicals and electric shock make their demands. CPR and advanced life support—typically called a "code"—have become so routine that it is expected to be done if there is no order *against* it. The patient's family can sue for negligence if it isn't, for failure to uphold the "standard of practice," to act prudently.

"The policy now is you have to code someone," says Bonnie. "If someone is a full code and you come in and they're not responsive, you have to code them. I asked the CPR instructor, 'Does that mean even if they're cold?' and she said yes." Bonnie has a strong dislike for emergencies, for the rush and the panic and the results.

"I was taught if you don't witness it, why bother? Way back when I was just getting out of high school, I worked as an aide. And people got sick and they died, or you'd go in there and see Mrs. So-and-so, ninety-eight years old, dead, and that was the end of it. You didn't dump them on the floor and start CPR.

"I was involved in two codes in one week's time on people that didn't have a no-code order, even though both had clearly stated that they didn't want that," says Erin Myers, the evening-shift nurse. "One of them died in the parking lot, with us beating on her chest. That, to me, is not the way to die." She is grimly amused at the idea. "I would hope that when *I* die, my last moments would be a calm easing out with somebody just being with me, not that horrible, horrible pounding on the chest and everything that surrounds it."

But problems arise, problems. For one thing, a lot of people in the medical establishment find the idea of an undelayed death much more horrible than the pounding, believing that the postponement is always in the patient's best interest. These are death haters, scared, afraid of their own shadow cast by a slowly falling sun. But this attitude and the gradual acceptance of electronic machinery at the bedside have given heroic life support a new cachet, such that when a person dies it only signals a new phase in treatment. It is as though we were all to be subjected to appendectomies at the age of ten just because the surgical technique had become so common. The dance of death becomes the dance of death prevention: our purpose to hinder and harry its course as long as possible, to kill, as it were, death itself.

This is where the living will enters. A living will is a document of uncertain legal status in which a person proclaims the desire to be allowed to die a natural death when death or a life of permanent coma—a life of "poor quality"—can't be prevented. Some living wills specify the treatments to be avoided: ventilators, codes, and so on. Others simply state the desire to avoid "heroic or extraordinary" measures, a category of considerable fluidity. Living wills are fine and good, but not enough: plenty of people on ventilators and feeding tubes have them. Susan Stevens has one, Conrad Berry has one—somewhere. Physicians are not, in most cases, legally obliged to uphold a living will. And living wills grow outdated, and must be rewritten, witnessed again, to have weight. As Paula Schulz points out, one doesn't usually file one with the nursing home in which one goes to die. By then it's too late. The uncertainty that surrounds the living will and the various "natural death" acts legislated in several states—and, of course, surrounded by confusion and disagreement—have led to a new vehicle, the "Durable Power of Attorney for Health Care." Like any power of attorney, it grants the right to make certain decisions about a person to a proxy. Its "durability" is reflected in the fact that it only becomes active after the person becomes incompetent, unable to act for himself. It is specific to health care. With the DPAHC a person in good health can designate another person to make critical health decisions in his or her place, and know the decisions will be legally binding. The power is enormous, and quite a thing to grant to another for ourselves. But we grant it every day, to hospitals, to physicians.

Even with such a potent document as the DPAHC, the bureaucracy and its slow, quotidian demands must be confronted. The physician is an integral part of that process, of instituting the documented desires of the comatose person in bed, or circumventing the lack of evidence of those desires. It is possible to get an order prohibiting a code; they are called no-code orders or DNRs, for "do not resuscitate." Harvest Moon has struggled with the problem of clarifying such orders for six years, and various unsatisfactory policies have been written. The efficacy—and the quality of the results—of CPR drops rapidly after a few minutes of oxygen deprivation. One of Harvest Moon's failed policies stated that on a patient who was considered a code, CPR would be done unless it was an "unwitnessed attack of longer than five minutes."

"What if the nurse is in the room and the patient's alive, and then she goes out and retrieves medicine from the cart and comes back in and the patient's not breathing? That's a witnessed attack," Paula Schulz explained. "But we know there are people who will say, 'Didn't see them go down, can't code them.' The new wording will be 'known to have occurred within the last five minutes.' That leaves them to *have to make a decision* and that's okay. That's what they're trained to do. Was it five minutes or was it seven? Maybe it was three. Well, make up your mind. Then, on the other hand, we had a patient who was probably down for ten minutes and they coded her."

All this brings to the forefront the specter of the "slow code," a desperate measure of nurses who *know*, either through conversation or experience, that a person doesn't want to be coded—as in the case of a woman whose daughter told Nancy Rice, "She's a hundred years old, I've buried her a thousand times. When she dies, let her go in peace." Without the formalization of such a wish on paper, doctor-approved, the nurse is obligated to do CPR. Hence the slow code. It is used, too—without a word, silently—in the difficult and murky times when a nurse believes, struggling, hurt, that the person should just be allowed to die because of the hopelessness of their condition. The slow code is just that—slow, preceded by a coffee break or a linen change in another room, not discussed, not documented, but a giving of time to a person rapidly becoming an unreachable corpse, oxygen-poor, never to be recovered. It is granted as a blessing and a grace, out of love.

One of the more bitter jokes in nursing circles is that of wearing a necklace—or better yet, a tattoo near the left breast—that says, NO CODE. Last year, as the head nurse in a large nursing home, I had to make a decision, a split-second one filled with regret, to code a woman in her nineties. I would never have considered doing it, but the woman happened to die while two of her children were visiting, and they felt a palpable and horror-struck shock. I explained—while she gurgled to death in the room beyond—what could be done, what its chances were, and they leaped for it, begging, please. So we did it, while they waited, and as I pressed on her thin and brittle ribs I felt them splinter into pieces, and when she threw up black vomit on me I wiped it away and kept going. The woman died—or rather, was deemed finally, irrevocably dead—in the hospital emergency room, and the children—themselves elderly—seemed to accept it, this second declaration from a white-coated physician, knowing, as they did, that everything possible had been done.

To avoid these memorable scenes means getting a DNR order from the physician—and preferably one supported by written consent from the patient or the family. Physicians vary widely in their reaction to such a request—from an easy yes without the slightest consultation with the family to a hurried no in spite of the family's wishes. Once a doctor told me to write—as his official order—"what the family wishes." His intention may have been a good one, but such a failure of decision paved the way for the worst of scenes, the frantic phone calls, the hurried explanation under pressure. Some physicians simply fail to note the obvious, assuming "everyone understands"; others just wish to avoid an uncomfortable conversation. It is left to the nurses to ferret out all the support they can, legal and otherwise, for what becomes more obvious to them every day.

Several months ago I called the physician of a ninety-year-old woman newly admitted to the nursing home where I worked part-time. She was recovering from a hip surgery and in apparently good health, but his orders failed to explain about CPR.

"What's the code status on this patient?" I asked.

"Oh, you won't have that problem," he replied.

That answer threw me a little. "Um, doctor, it's never a problem until it happens. She *is* ninety years old."

"Look," he answered, impatient now, "this woman doesn't have a single lethal condition—"

"Except old age," I interrupted, impatient as well.

"Except old age, but don't worry about it," he said. "She's not going to die."

"Doctor, I have to have a code status on every patient," I

said, trying a new tack. I was tired, by then, of such talk from someone who is never around when the person dies.

"Okay, then," he answered, thoroughly exasperated. "I guess you should give her the works."

"Most of the nurses, when someone goes sour, you can pretty much go in and look at someone and you kinda get this feeling—that they're not doing very well—a lot of the times you'll get them into the emergency room, or get hold of the doctor and let him know. And sometimes the code status is just obtained in a very short time," says Bonnie Pereira. "There are a couple on C Wing right now that are obviously DNRs, but it wasn't carried through on the orders." Such mistakes of omission are never any one person's fault, but the fault of a forgetful doctor, overworked nurse, too many phone calls passing information, no extra minutes to catch up with business.

"We always kid the night nurses—they get two or three deaths in a few shifts and we say, 'Now you put that pillow back in the closet.' " This was one of Paula's black jokes when we talked about deaths in December. But she's gone today; she had that funeral to attend.

For years the ventilator was the central concern—the plug to be pulled. But now it's the feeding tube. A ventilator is somehow more obvious, more enormously invasive than a small plastic feeding tube. It is big and complicated and has a palpable purpose, instantaneous and constant. It is the breath and the air, every few seconds. The most medically ignorant person can watch a ventilator breathe for someone and know what turning off the machine will mean—and mean immediately, not a few days or weeks later. The last breath of the ventilator is also the last breath of the ventilated. There is a kind of relief in that one, and final, exhalation.

Feeding tubes don't share this sense of immediacy. We eat now and again, survive missed meals with only minor discomfort. We know this in our primitive selves, our hunter-gatherer guts. In fact, we're culturally trained to consider food a case of too much, not too little, something to control. We are untrained to feel hunger, and the idea of starvation is a foreign and distant one. One never starves *right now*, but without a feeding tube or other, even more aggressive treatment, a comatose person will certainly starve in a week or two—and likely die of thirst before that. Not only is the feeding tube less obviously vital than the ventilator, its loss is less immediately apparent—the death that results slower, and more prolonged. Yet many physicians and nurses find it more difficult to turn off the ventilator—that big breathing *thing,* so important—than to remove a tube, a little, simple plastic tube.

Talking about feeding tubes in terms of starvation is discouraged. It is a harsh and dangerous word, a word for propaganda. But Phoebe White tried, till she lost interest, to starve herself last October, and in the spring of 1986 the American Medical Association, a body not known for its radical departures from standards, adopted a policy that categorized artificial methods of nourishment, like feeding tubes, as extraordinary life support. The AMA encouraged its members to use discretion and forethought, to be motivated by the desire to alleviate suffering first of all. A number of higher courts have agreed, in principle, and allowed family members to discontinue nourishment to comatose relatives. (Other courts have refused; precedents are contradictory. The point I find odd is how often the courts have refused such a choice to the patient himself when he is cognizant and alert, and making his own request. There are many such cases on record; the middle-aged woman with Lou Gehrig's disease, a wasting illness like multiple sclerosis, the young woman with severe cerebral palsy, the quadriplegic man—each told that because of their clear minds, they were doomed to live. The logic appears to be that a clear mind creates a higher quality of life, and thus a greater need to hold on to that life, than a lost or clouded mind—even when the clarity is one of absolute dependence and pain. To be unaware of one's condition is a step toward being removed from it.)

To Paula the feeding tube, though different from Erin Myers's "horrible, horrible pounding," is violence nonetheless. "Is an NG tube down your nose with stuff being poured into your stomach *natural*? Normal? You put a catheter in for comfort, you inject pain medication for comfort, not as life-sustaining procedures. An NG tube is." Paula has always been free with these ideas, and vocal. She is in a position to see quite a large part of the picture: the patient's condition, the family's desires, the physician's concerns. "The biggest thing I always fall back on is when a family comes to me and says, 'My mother told me not to *ever* put her in a nursing home and keep her alive, and that's exactly what I'm doing. If she could get out of bed right now, she'd be furious with me.' When I know that a patient felt *that* strongly about it, and now the whole process is out of their hands, out of control—that we're doing all this against their wishes, man, I don't have a problem with stopping it. When you have to fight to put a tube down, aren't you violat-ing their rights at every level? Unless you've been declared in-competent by a court of law, you're still considered competent, I don't care *how* unconscious you may be."

Harvest Moon is bound to offer food and fluids to every pa-tient a certain number of times a day. But what is appropriate for a person who can't swallow? There are many options. Needles in the vein, which never last for long, are delicate, painful. The traditional feeding tube is called an NG for "nasogastric," or nose-to-stomach. A tube can also be permanently inserted into the stomach through a hole, or stoma, made in the abdominal wall, called a gastrostomy. Susan Stevens has been offered gastrostomy, and she refuses; her NG tube dislodges and plugs up frequently, and the process of replacing it is painful and dis-concerting, and a little dangerous because of her spasming throat muscles and gritting teeth—a deft hand is required to avoid the bronchial tubes, the lungs, and aspiration pneumonia.

There are new high-tech tricks for the alert and oriented patient, the educable—hyperalimentation, a complete form of nutrition fed directly into the bloodstream. The details grow more refined every day. Eating itself grows almost obsolete.

Paula has an old-fashioned method she pulls out of her bag of tricks from time to time. Called clysis, it is the insertion of an I.V. needle not in a vein, but into a muscle, which gradually absorbs the slow drip of fluid. Clysis by itself won't normally keep a person alive, but is thought to ease the discomfort of thirst.

All this rigmarole comes to one point: sometimes tubes are pulled. Sometimes Paula and the responsible family members reach that mutual choice, having never had a chance to reach the original choice together.

Talking about Susan Stevens, the young multiple sclerosis patient, and her long wait for death, Paula quoted Susan's doctor: "He said you have to hire some bad nurses over there—you give *too* good nursing care." *That's* what produces the question of taking out the tube, because we can keep them alive for so long that the family can't deal with it emotionally, financially, they just *can't go on.* But you also have to remember the guilt so many families feel when they give permission to have that tube put down and then they realize what it's going to mean, that the person will go on forever, that they took it out of the hands of God. A lot of soul-searching goes on with those people before they even approach you and say, 'Is there even a possibility that we could talk about this?' And they're usually very surprised that they can talk about it and accept it and we'll continue to give the patient good care, whether the tube is in or not."

So the tube is pulled. It's a simple procedure, takes only a few moments. Who can judge the subjective experience of the comatose? We have only our own comfort, our own imagination, to consider. Feeding tubes and clysis, aspirin to lower fevers and even the catheter, for comfort—hard to say how much

152

is appreciated, how much ignored. But we have to judge it somehow, have to *guess*—we haven't anything else to go on. But, though we ourselves grow desperate for that final relieved exhalation from the lover or parent in bed, almost everyone cringes at the idea, when it is directly confronted, of a person dying of thirst.

Paula points out that she never withholds food and water, or what is more euphemistically, distantly, called nutrition and hydration. It is always offered. But this might mean holding a cup to the lips of an unconscious person, knowing full well they can't drink. Barbie Moscowitz, a few weeks before she quit, said, "Withholding nutrition does not bother me, if everything is documented well, it's well planned, it's been discussed, the doctor's been straightforward with the family. But it bothers me greatly if they withhold hydration. I just know what *I* feel, what I've heard and seen and what I've felt when I was dehydrated. I think you need to consider that whether a person is in a coma or not. All I think we can judge by is what physically happens when you do these things to people." Barbie is concerned with suffering, the easing of pain. Which is more painful, the week of thirst or the months in a coma?

My friend who runs the nursing home with so many problems just told me a story, with a story inside it. An elderly man admitted his wife to the facility. She was in a deep coma from a stroke that had destroyed all but the most primitive parts of her brain. She was fed by a tube, and a few days after her admission the family and physician decided to remove the tube. The tube came out on a Sunday, when my friend was off work. She had a little difficulty with that, because of the problem with thirst—and sure enough, when she went to the woman's husband with her concerns, he admitted that he was taken aback, that he hadn't realized she would get no water, either. They agreed to have the tube put back in to allow a small amount of water every day. It spared, before he knew of it, the old grieving man another difficulty, perhaps a sadder one. Without the feeding tube the woman would have had to be moved to another wing, because she would lose her Medicare coverage and no longer qualify for skilled care. The nursing home's tight budget had no room for a few charity weeks in that lucrative section. The woman would have gone to the intermediate-care wing, to a new room, to new nurses and aides, lower staffing ratios, and more distractions. The woman died a short time later, apparently in peace, and my friend just shuffles her pile of Medicare reports and fee schedules and shakes her head.

All this raises one last, painful question. If we are easing, ever so slowly and cautiously, to the admission that it is all right to allow a person to die—to withhold, if necessary, even food in order to accomplish that—then why don't we leap beyond? Withholding food is passive euthanasia, the same as withholding insulin from a diabetic or antibiotics from a person with pneumonia. Why don't we look each other in the eye, agree to be done with this verbiage, and prepare a large syringe of morphine? Is it just because the one requires action, deliberation, and the other merely the willingness to wait? Where do we begin to slide down that "slippery slope"—if one really exists—into barbarism and genocide? Not long ago I suggested, on a late-night radio talk show, that there are times when a terminally ill person should be allowed to die, should not be force-fed. I was careful to balance my remarks, fall far from radical suggestions. And a few minutes later a woman called up, quoted Adolf Hitler, compared me to a Nazi, that I should imagine such a thing, that I could be so cold.

In the end it is our own discomfort that we try to soothe. I came to visit Cecil Lunt this morning and found him even more placid, more distant, than before. His nurse told me, "I don't like the way he looks these last few days." She said it with sincere concern, with worry. What is she really saying? Does she really *worry* that he might die, fear it, feel it would be an unfortunate thing? What do the deaths of these patients, so nearly lost to us already, so poised between, really mean? We grow so unaccountably fond of them; they are so unknowingly dependent on us. We worry and fret over their declines for a long time, exuding the sorrows of their long loss and the nature of its going—and still feel an inexplicable loss of our own when they finally go. Perhaps it is in their awful sameness, the brutal predictability of their demise, that we seek something unique— the individual—and, finding it in quiet days and restless nights beside them, feel the taking of it more acutely for the difficulty in the search.

Certainly the subjective experience of the woman who died in the parking lot wasn't what any of us would seek. But then, neither is that of the man on his back, lungs pumped by a machine. The individual patient's experience hasn't always been a concern to doctors battling disease, but for the nurses willing to care for a patient while he starves to death it is, ironically, the greatest concern of all. It is to prevent suffering that we pull the tube, to spare the helpless not-a-stranger under our hands more pain, a more difficult death. Erin Myers calls feeding tubes "an exercise in futility"; she shakes her head each time another such person is admitted. Here we go again, she thinks, into another prolonged and unimagined future.

"I was born and raised on a farm and when an animal was suffering or maimed you put it out of its misery," says John Eldizondo. He feels it as a conviction and sorrow. "It's too bad we can't do that with people. I think it should be done sometimes. I think about Gerry Kennett, used to hanging by now.

"Some people think I'm a bit of a cold-blooded sucker because I don't get sad and cry when people die. I used to be a softhearted kid and cry. My mother, when little chicks would die, you know, she'd just cover them up in the bedding until nighttime, after I'd gone to bed. Then she'd throw the little dead ones out. She couldn't do it during the day, I'd just be crying all day long."

He holds his big body carefully on the edge of the chair, his hands flat on his huge thighs like a farmer in church. It is as though he has to hold on to his own strength in order to control it. He keeps it in reserve, till it's required. John remembers, soft-voiced, almost nostalgic, his first sight of Vietnam: "We went flying in there and saw the green on the ground and I was thinking what a pretty place it was—like Arkansas or something.

"Vietnam was a nightmare. And I think something happened in my childhood with dying animals and all that stuff. I've gotten calluses around my soft heart."

CHAPTER TWELVE

Chaos

Leon Poretz has Martin King, the physical therapist, pinned, back to the nurses' desk, hands at his side. Martin in his amiability has become a captive audience; there is no telling when Leon will allow him to go. Leon Poretz is eighty-five years old and still active in the business he began as an entrepreneur decades ago. He is recovering from a stroke and increasing problems with a lung disease which recently put him to bed—first in the hospital and now at Harvest Moon—for several weeks. Now that it is almost time for his discharge, he must apply to renew his driver's license.

"Now, will you call that doctor? Mr. King, I need your help," he implores. He is several inches shorter than Martin, intense, a rooster.

"I'll see what I can do," answers Martin, politely. He turns to go, but Leon puts up an arm.

"I gotta drive, Mr. King," he says. "I got things I gotta do."

In an earlier care conference Margery Todd had laughed at Poretz's insistence on a license. His chronic illnesses and long recoveries have made it difficult for him to handle finances and created problems for his work—and those problems in turn are increasing his anxiety and concern. He refuses Nancy's suggestion of a retirement home—"He'd be perfect for it, if we could just get him there," she said. "He's wonderful. He's feisty and he's going to get out of here, and he's going to drive." She shook her head, still laughing. "Of course, we'll all stay off the road if we can figure out when he's *on* it."

She laughs, but the truth is that when Leon Poretz goes home, almost no one at Harvest Moon will know what becomes of him, unless he returns. Nancy Rice has time for the plan and the process of discharge, but almost none for followup. Now and then a staff member will grow so attached to a patient that he or she continues to call or drop by long after the patient has returned home. Sometimes the family or the patient himself stays in touch, through cards, donations, or Christmas presents, but all these gestures fade with time. Harvest Moon exists in a certain place in time for its residents, and after they go it ceases to exist in a very important way. And for those who remain, the community at hand is far more absorbing, more immediate. Only people like me, not quite a part, have the leisure of both time and mental space to satisfy their curiosity.

Annie Brun, who had "a real good time" while recovering from her stroke at Harvest Moon, is back in her own home. She greeted me at the door yesterday, after a delay of several minutes, behind a cumbersome walker. Her little white dog yipped all around her feet, until she lowered herself gratefully into a wheelchair. Then the dog jumped into her lap and barked at me with glee.

"I get tired real easy," she smiled, happy to have a visitor. Her daughter and grandchildren live in the basement apartment of her large ranch-style house in the suburbs. A widow, Annie lives alone in the main part of the house. "I can't walk real well yet," she said. "And I'm a pianist and an organist, and I haven't been able to do that." She pointed at the far end of the long living room, where a baby grand piano and full-size organ stood, shiny, dust-free. She and her husband had been music teachers and musicians together during their long marriage. "Oh, well, I did that for sixty years, now I'll do something else. I think I might tell my autobiography into a tape recorder. For my grandkids, you know. I don't know if anyone else would be interested." She asked me to get her a glass of water and a sweater, then added, "I want to take swimming lessons, too. That's something I never did. And get my hair done."

"My fanny's sore," says Margaret Bond, still at Harvest Moon. She is no better; her hip refuses to stay where it belongs, and each X ray of the joint shows it looking more vulnerable, flimsier. She's been off her feet for over three months now, fending off the blunting boredom with game shows and newspapers and long chats. Her husband visits every day; they sit near each other in the dining room and share the pages of a two-day-old newspaper.

More news, and it all takes on a dry tone, a list of facts: she's better, he died, they fired her. Custer Holland has gone home, leaving behind him a surprised and pleased Martin King. He left walking, tall and unbowed, resolute. Gerry Kennett has been seen more. Once or twice a week she has let herself be propped in a wheelchair, tube neatly pinned behind her, as discreet as such a thing can be, and wheeled down the hall. She sits with a dignified expression on her face, seeing and being seen.

Gertrude Werner, dependable Gertrude, has her pants rolled up to the knee with care, loose bobby socks several inches below an expanse of naked calf. Gina Tyrell sees her thus exposed as she heads past the physical therapy door to the dining room, and calls after her.

"Now what you want your pants like that for?"

Gertrude turns to look at her with exaggerated deliberation, stares, and then turns back down her road.

Gina follows her down the hall and stops her with a word. She points to the pants, bends down to unroll them. Gertrude protests, wordlessly, waving her hands. The discussion continues for a few minutes, and then Gina gives up, standing straight again.

"Well, okay baby," she says as she walks back to the desk. "Take it easy, baby."

Under the birdcage a few yards away two janitors lean against the wall, heads together. They are both dark-skinned, dark-haired, with suspicious smiles. They watch each person pass by, conspiratorial. A woman in a calf-length fur coat sways past, heading for the street door, and as she turns the corner one man elbows the other in the ribs.

"Yo, Rafael!" he says in a stage whisper. "Lookit that! A lotta little animals died to make *that!*"

And while these minor plays unfold onstage, the machinations of the stagehands unfold, too. Harvest Moon will computerize. The accounting and medical records departments have used computers for years, but Roger Scarpelli has announced a plan to add fourteen small personal computer stations throughout the facility—at the nurses' desk, by the receptionist, in the therapy departments. All patient information, statistics, medical test results, and billing and personnel records will be compiled and held in the computer. Roger projects a target date of mid-February, realizing that certain "adjustments" must be made: there is no room at the nurses' desk for *anything* new, let alone a computer station. The reception area is unguarded, insecure. But these are minor problems, easily solved with a little construction and patience. The system will cost "over a hundred thousand dollars," according to Roger. The savings in labor, the increased efficiency, are expected to pay its way. Now Roger is beginning to read about robotics, computerized lifts and labor-saving devices for washing patients, serving food. He dreams, and gazes out his big picture window to the parking lot, the hedge beyond.

While Roger dreams, Willie washes dishes, breakfast and lunch. He is Willie the dishwasher, known to all, free with a pat on the arm—or bottom—and a laugh. I walked through the kitchen a while back and found him singing to himself as he mopped the floor in the dishwashing alcove. "The heart of rock 'n' roll's still *beating*," he warbled, bending over the mop in rhythm, swaying to his own time.

He rinses, washes, sterilizes, and dries the flatware, cups, and plates; washes down the food carts, takes out the garbage, and mops the floor.

"That's not part of my job, you know," he says of the mopping. "I don't have to do that. I just do it 'cause it's nice, you know."

Willie is thirty-seven years old. He stands five feet tall and has a rotund belly circling his belt. He has a round, soft, brown face with dark eyes and soft dark hair, and at the bottom of that circle has a little mouth, lips almost puckered. He was trained as a counselor after majoring in political science, and worked for years with drug addicts, veterans, and teenagers. And then, inexplicably, he moved thousands of miles away from his native Hawaii and took a job as a dishwasher at Harvest Moon, almost a year ago.

"This is a good job, you know. It keeps me busy. It's not boring. It keeps me off the street, I guess." He works constantly, talking at the same speed. He takes a tray covered with trash and food out of the laden food cart and methodically, rapidly, dumps the leftover food down a giant garbage disposal, pours the liquids from cups down a drain, then stacks the cups, glasses, and plates in separate trays. It takes almost two hours to clean up the debris from breakfast.

He is president of a local club for Pacific island natives. "My friends there, they ask me, 'What do you do with your time?' And I say I wash pots and pans in a nursing home, and they say, '*What?* Holy cow, why do you wanna do that?' I say, 'It's a good job, you should try it.' " Willie is meticulous, almost finicky in his cleaning. He refuses to wear an apron, claiming that he is so careful he never soils his clothes. He claims, too, to be quite happy here, to be particularly comfortable in the company of old women.

"Hey, you know, I got a mother, she's seventy-six. She's not like these people, she still works." He spends coffee breaks and lunch hours in the dining room with patients, sharing coffee. Now and then he barrels through the double doors from the kitchen to the hallway, carrying a treat for a particularly picky resident. It is Willie's special duty to coax food down reluctant mouths.

"They always pass away, you know. Since I've worked here all my favorites have passed away." He slips a filled tray into the sterilizer. "One thing that really bothers me is the waste," he says, dropping most of a meal in the disposal. "Look at all this, all this waste! Sometimes there's whole trays that aren't touched! And there's people out there starving, just starving. But I'm used to it now. It depends on what mood they're in. One day they like chicken, the next day they don't. You never know.

"You can tell if the nurse's aide is in a good mood because the cart is clean. If it's dirty—oh, sometimes it's filthy. And I go out there and tell the nurses, you better have a talk with your aide, this cart is filthy. There's no excuse for that." He wrinkles his nose. "And I go talk to the director, I don't care. They don't have to like me. They're all my friends, they don't have to like me."

He leans out the double doors that meet with a swish of rubber, glancing suspiciously around the dining room, planning his break. He sees Phoebe White in the middle of the room, alone at a long, empty table, facing the west bank of windows. He winks, and ducks back into the kitchen. "She's trouble. You want trouble, you get Phoebe. Put her next to Maude Davis, they'll kill each other," he smiles, admonition in his voice.

He keeps hard hours, arriving between four and five in the

morning and leaving early in the afternoon. In slack times he makes sandwiches to put in the vending machine in the dining room, or mops again. "I can't work nights! I'm single, I gotta have a social life." Several times he's come to work without sleep. He rolls his eyes to the kitchen where Doris Garland and her silent helpers prepare dinner. "These people, they all about as old as my mother. They don't party here." He dances a jig between cart and sink, humming.

Phoebe has trouble of her own. Later I leave Willie, contentedly fiddling with a steam vent, and wander through stuffy halls, rustling with rushes of cold winter air, to find her. I am growing fond of Phoebe White, who is more confused each time I see her. She retains the genteel concern with propriety, struggling to make each exchange correct, long past remembering the purpose of correctness. She is growing sadder. Last week she wandered down the hallway in tears, angry because she didn't recognize her "maid," the young female aide who seemed an inexplicable stranger. Addie, the therapy assistant, leaned over her chair: "What's wrong?" she asked, solicitous, maternal. "I'm frightened," whined Phoebe, so young. "Of what?" "I don't *know!*" said Phoebe, and the tears poured out, as Addie steered her to her room, brought her hot tea, held her hand. When Phoebe sees me today—and I know she doesn't know me, is past learning who I am no matter how many times we meet—she immediately starts to cry, alone in her darkened room with a table of Christmas cards spread before her.

"I don't know what to do, I just *don't know what to do,*" she tells me, and tears fall. "It's a sorry world."

I still feel guilty when my presence makes a person cry, even though years of conversation with confused older people has taught me better. It isn't *my* presence that makes Phoebe cry today, a grim cold winter day—it is my *presence,* and for that I've no need to be sorry at all. Without my presence, without a human voice, a hand, a touch, her pain would have no focus, and then perhaps no tears (does a tree falling . . . ?)—but maybe in the focus is a purge. I don't really know, and her grief surprises me today, catches me off guard.

She pulls me down, kisses first one cheek, then another, grips a hand so I won't turn and go.

"I'm lonely, lonely." And I see almost immediately that the force of emotion itself is taking her out of the relentless, undirected sorrow. It is taking her, and almost as a blessing, to the surf of dementia again, lost in words and an almost pleasant ignorance in which she can rest again in the arms of others.

"They just say, say, are you in or, and I say, why, I don't know, I don't know what I'm supposed to do. So they, you know." And so she goes, calmer now, more interested in the answer she'll never find instead of the question she can't formulate.

Chaos itself is a shifting thing: the jabber of Max Kleiner and the bewildered noblesse oblige of Phoebe White seem utterly chaotic to one unused to them. On the rare occasions when I am around heavy machinery I feel the same stricken anxiety, small and vulnerable in the midst of noise and smell and chuttering vibrations I can't identify, wondering which signal disaster, which rescue. Perhaps it is the gradual awakening of chaos into order that is the heart of familiarity, of coming to terms with what we fear. Standing at the intersection of hallways, I can see it almost as a braid, plaited half by luck and half by talent, in which the differently colored strands combine into another, unexpected shade. I see it as a braid, and someone else sees it as a nightmare of derangement. I feel surprised that such an intricate braid is made at all, and another feels it as a blow to the head. These are tenuous contracts we make with each other; the braid isn't tightly woven, entropy lurks in file cabinets and closets, the curve is always toward chaos, dirt, and waste, poverty and powerlessness.

Behind the nurses' desk, between the two bulky scales and the storage room, is the housekeeping bulletin board. The housekeepers and janitors hold themselves apart, socializing a bit with each other but rarely with the nursing staff or administration. It is a job burdened by infinity, by endlessness, and by a kind of invisibility. The housekeepers are expected to be there, to clean up spills and move along, without comment. The janitors trail wires out of wall sockets, open mysterious closets filled with pipes, and move along. I see them glance up at activity nearby, turn to a sound, and then look back at each other and keep working.

There are rules and memos all over the bulletin board, written in careful block letters and posted there by Phyllis Johnson, the housekeeping supervisor for the past five years. "Keep top of closets cleaned off," reads one. "Soiled mop head [sic] go in yellow linen barrels," reads another. And at the bottom of the page, "TB test given before new employee's [sic] can start must have result back." Phyllis lectures too; last week she gave a class on "safety prevention."

She looks, at forty-eight, as though she'd bitten off a piece tougher to chew than she'd expected—a little surprised, and shopworn. Phyllis takes considerable pride in her work, a personal pride, and pulls the little immigrant girls who fill her ranks to her heart, teaching them small phrases of English, new skills, survival in a world of too few jobs.

"I take pride in the compliments we get from visitors, families, friends—there's no odor, the floor's looking nice and shiny," she says. "It may not seem much to you, but it does to me. The group of people we have working for us does a bang-up job, as far as I'm concerned. And you meet people. It's nice to see a patient get well and go home and see the smile on their faces. And we have a bang-up physical therapy department, too, real good.

"We're lowest on the totem pole," she adds. "There's all different types of personalities, like they wouldn't bother picking up a mop. They would call housekeeping to do it, they feel it would be below them to wipe up a spill. And it doesn't take two seconds to mop it up."

Certain superficial notions of who has power and who does not rule daily life. There are, of course, many different kinds of power, some more desirable than others. The visible life at Harvest Moon is a putting to rights, scurrying labor bent toward repair. Broken things are fixed, separate raw ingredients skillfully blended. The linen and dirty dressings go over the shoulder and into the can, the coffee cup is left on the counter and forgotten. The patient, poor fellow, has better things to think about. But what is dirty must be made clean, and, in the same peculiar pattern repeated a world and history over, it is the lowliest labor of all, and perhaps the most important.

The housekeepers are so present it is easy to miss them. They slip into rooms and shy away, a bit skittish. But when the nurses are gone, the housekeepers open a little, at home more with the old women and men in their beds than with the white-suited professionals nearby. In this way they share with the aides a particular privilege, little noted: it is the product of close, daily contact with the most powerless group of all, the patients. There is a sense of separation at work—but not one of quality. It is a difference of purpose again, a separation in intent and goal.

Several months ago Harvest Moon had an epidemic of scabies, a tiny mite that burrows under the skin and lays eggs—an itching infestation, easily spread, uncomfortable in the extreme. At first the patients affected—thirteen—were treated singly, with the hot baths and medicated skin ointment necessary. But the infection kept growing, and finally Janet Krause organized, with Phyllis's help, a two-day shakedown. Ordinary activities were suspended, employees called in on their day off. The ninety-eight people in residence were each bathed with medicated shampoo. Each room, from curtain to bedframe, was disinfected. Each mattress was disinfected separately. All the linen, all the personal clothes, were washed. And it worked.

"Everybody chipped in," recalls Phyllis. It was one of her golden moments, a tour de force of organization. "Paula Schulz got in there and cleaned a couple of rooms. That made us feel good, too, kind of boosted our ego. If she can get down there and work, then we don't mind doing it. She was not proud. It shocked some of them to see her in there in her little gown, scrubbing. The people that seen her in there, it made them feel, 'Well, look who's here.'

"We go and get 'em coffee, a tissue or something," says Phyllis of the patients. The housekeepers are strictly forbidden to touch a patient, because of insurance coverage. "I have found not to get too close to a person, but sometimes I do. It hurts me the most when you have holidays, Mother's Day, and the kids don't show up. And I can feel it, and I'm not even that person. Couldn't they take five minutes to call, a few hours to come down?" Phyllis shakes her head. "Just to see Mom? You'd be surprised how many times it doesn't happen. I guess the world is self-centered."

"They look forward to seeing me every morning. Makes me feel good, when I come to work. Like if y'all are off for a coupla days and you come back and they be waving and stuff like that. They glad I'm back. Make *me* feel important."

Alice has been a housekeeper at Harvest Moon for nearly a year. She is "more than thirty-five," plump and pretty, neatly coiffed and clean. She straightens her hair into a small bun behind her smooth face.

"I mop and do garbage cans and polish chromes on the bed, wash windowsills. I wash windows about once a week. I *hate* windows. There's things we don't have to do, but if I have time to do I can.

"The only thing I can't stand is, they wish I was a nurse. At first I thought I would like that work but now I think I'd rather just housekeep. I come in and ask 'em how they doing, 'bout going home, they shows me pictures on the wall, ask me do I have children. When I been away a while some of the ones on my wing might've passed away that got sick. I love ever'body on B Wing."

167

She is a widow with several teenage children and one, twenty-two, who's returned from military duty to live at home again. "Lord, they can eat! I get Social Security checks. It would be hard if this was the only income I had. I couldn't make it.

"I don't really have anything else to do. I have a boyfriend but he's not there all the time, neither. This gives me something to do. Coming here, it doesn't bother me. I think, I *get* to go to work, tell you the truth."

There is almost a competition for the lowest rung, for the self-justification of others' disrespect. Like the aides, proud of their labors done almost in secret, the housekeepers keep a silent tally—not bitter, but rather smug in the knowledge of credit earned but not yet spent.

Harvest Moon has a basement. It can only be reached by going outside into the parking lot and down two flights of concrete stairs, open to the weather. The walls in the basement are concrete, like the floor. The ceiling is high above your head, to accommodate the two huge gas dryers that never cease their roar. Five days a week three people—two aides and their supervisor—work here from seven in the morning till half past three. On the weekends two aides work the same shift, alone.

"As soon as we get here in the morning we start to fold. We used to have a night person for four hours but as soon as Roger got here he stopped that."

Shirley is the supervisor, a white-haired woman in her fifties who worked twenty years in retail stores before coming to Harvest Moon. The two aides folding towels on the table nearby are as similar as twin sisters: enormously fat, with dark brown hair pulled tightly back from faces young with extra flesh. They smoke while they work, the smoke drifting around their faces and swirling in the patterns of air formed by the endless folding of linen. One of the aides, Lucy, talks, the other listens. Both have worked here in the laundry for five years, and each makes $4.40 an hour.

Every load of laundry weighs forty pounds and they wash thirty-six loads every day. The carts are brought from the hallways to the dumbwaiter by the nurses' aides, who drop it and leave. The laundry staff separates it, loads the various groupings into the wash, moves it to the dryer, carries it to the folding table, and then folds, counts, and stacks the clean laundry back onto the carts. Clean carts go up three times a day, usually steered by Shirley, who must then put the various piles away in their proper places. The laundry also washes the personal clothes of the residents, according to individual specifications, and must count everything they wash: yesterday it included 133 hospital gowns, 147 towels, 525 washcloths, and almost 100 sheets. They mend personal clothes and return them to the individual closets; sweep and mop the cold floors of the laundry, and take out the garbage.

"We're always running out of linen. Don't ask me where it disappears to, but it does," says Shirley.

Lucy snorts. "Nursing throws away our washcloths and then complains to us that they don't have enough. They throw people's clothes in the barrel, and they don't have names on them, so they never get back where they belong."

The basement is cold in the winter and hot in the summer. A few small windows are perched at ground level, shielded by uncut grass. The machines fill the room with a multitude of ocean sounds, metallic bumps and whines. There is no bathroom here; to find one the staff must go outside, climb the stairs, and walk around the building to the bathroom near the receptionist's desk inside.

"We never get recognized down here," says Shirley, smoking, patient. "They always forget about us. On Thanksgiving, when everybody gets fed free, they forgot to invite us. Only when they want a donation—then they always remember us. No one ever comes to visit." I doubt it has ever occurred to Shirley and her staff, but I can well imagine the result if the laundry aides decided to protest, if even one day passed without laundry service.

"People would care more if they made more than peanuts," says Lucy. Her friend nods silently. "I hear people say, if they're only going to pay us a little, I'm only going to give a little." Her hands are red and dry; she keeps folding. So few options. A certain misery cannot be spared, to the patients, to the workers who have no place to go, no better choice. There isn't so much difference between these groups, I think. I feel conscious of a world of choice offered me for no reason other than the luck of a middle-class birth. Without my goodwill, the goodwill of everyone with such luck, the unlucky have no safety. And our goodwill is always dependent on our own security, however we name it; it is offered only when we aren't in danger for the offering.

The walls are covered with posters: five different full-length photos of Michael Jackson, two Garfield cartoons, and jokes on plaques. Above Shirley's desk is a calendar of muscular young men in skimpy swimsuits.

"We all think April is the best-looking," she says.

CHAPTER THIRTEEN

Giving Way

Anna Rosenbaum still has a sore tongue. It lies in her mouth like a misbehaving pet, refusing to obey the simplest commands. She refuses to wear her dentures. Of more immediate concern—though less demanding of her attention, for she worries the tongue endlessly, rolling and fingering it—are her hips. There is nothing left to pin together, nothing to lean on for support. She is so thin that when she sits in her wheelchair there seems to be a foot of space on either side of her. Anna's legs twist awkwardly backward, away from the footrests. The few steps she takes, leaning on the arms of others, cost her great pain.

Nancy Rice says sadly that Anna has "met her potential." She shows no further chance of improvement or, in the nomenclature of payments, "rehabilitation." Harvest Moon has no vacancies on B and D wings, no place to keep another welfare patient with promised years of life left. Nancy has informed Anna she must transfer to another place in less than a week, back to a small ICF where she stayed briefly last year.

She pretends to crankiness. "How can I pack my stuff? I ain't got nobody to help. I ain't got any boxes. I don't even know where my clothes are," she tells me, and then repents. "Ah, siddown, honey. See my tongue? It's terrible."

Alone in the big three-bed ward, she admits a bleak loneliness. "I'm crippled. I ain't got nobody," she says quietly, her voice mumbling through the painful tongue. "It's no way to live, I tell ya. I wish the Good Lord would just take me away." When she goes this time I will never see her again—I could, I know where she's going. But Anna is leaving, this place, my life, and I can't race after her—so many people to follow, to leave.

Bonnie Pereira is thinking of leaving. "It's not official or anything," she says. "No one knows. But for the first time I'm starting to think about it. It's too much, too hard. I don't know if I can do it any more."

And Erin Myers, too. "I would not have stayed here five years if there wasn't something good about it. I'm probably in a rut—it's easier to stay than make a change." She looks tired, heavy, older than her twenty-eight years. "I think I might like to be a writer. I got derailed from going into journalism and got pushed into nursing a long time ago." But she has an investment, a big investment of time and money and emotion in nursing; she doubts she'll ever leave it completely. It is an easy job in one way—there is always work, the pay is enough. But where else could she go? "Hospitals—no, I don't like the attitude that they are so much better than we are here. You're branded, once you've been in a place like this. My idea of hospital nursing is very much oriented toward the saving of life, and I feel much more comfortable with the feeling we have here, of making people comfortable till the time of their death." But Erin wants to qualify that: "When it comes time to put my grandmother in a nursing home, there's no way I'd put her here. I look at those ICF wings and that's no kind of life."

Laura Lembke died in her sleep last night. She is the seventh person to die in January.

When I arrived early this morning the parking lot was almost full. Before ten a crowd had gathered in the dining room around the big color television usually reserved for soap operas and basketball games. Mike Wallace shakes his head in a mist of fuzzy yellow, the tube old and needing repair. He solemnly repeats himself as the same brief film clip is shown again and again: the space shuttle rises on a masterful course, compelling in its confidence, then seems to stutter in midflight, stumble as though over a rock hidden in the bright blue sky. The small pieces pause, then tumble end over end, all authority gone. We watch in silence a rumbling thunder we can't hear. I find myself crying, embarrassed, and looking around see Nancy Rice and Margery Todd crying, Buddy Mullin transfixed by the repeating image. Margaret Bond rattles her newspaper and says aloud, "Just like watching Kennedy get killed." Down the end of the dining room an aide leans over Gertrude Werner, who watches the group by the television with worry. The aide tells her, very loudly, "It's about a big ship that blew up." The usually silent laundry aide stands on the perimeter of the group. "You couldn't get *me* up in one o' them things," she says, to no one in particular.

A while later another small group forms, bent on errands, pausing over the nurses' desk to share the morbid disbelief that surrounds catastrophe. Paula Schulz leans on a pile of charts, talking to Ed Lewton, the pharmacist. They share the question that comes first to mind with losses both immediate and impersonal, the skeleton we pin it on in order to frame it in memory: Where were you when you heard? The shower, driving, breakfast, people answer. Ed and Paula start arguing about the day of the week John Kennedy was killed.

"I remember it was a Sunday, because I was in the hospital having Lindy," says Paula. "I woke up after she was born and my friend was there and she said, 'Did you hear Kennedy was shot?' And I said, '*That's* not funny.' "

But Ed disagrees, and reaches across the charts to grab the Yellow Pages, flipping until he finds the perpetual calendar buried inside. He is a large and myopic man, who has a habit of peering amiably about himself as he works through his requests. Now he is preoccupied with the problem at hand.

"See? November 22, 1963. It was a Friday." He is mildly triumphant.

Where were you when Neil Armstrong walked on the moon, when Richard Nixon resigned? It takes me a moment to realize how young all this history is, how naïve we are in the wisdom of experience. Phoebe White was already alive when X rays were discovered, when the Klondike gold rush began. As a child, Max Kleiner read of the Titanic sinking, the Wright brothers flying. When Anna Rosenbaum was my age, Sacco and Vanzetti were found guilty, and Albert Einstein won the Nobel Prize. In her life Maude Davis stared at photos of the Hindenburg exploding, read with shaking hands of the stock market crash, heard of the attack on Pearl Harbor in the shower, driving, at breakfast. A ship of dreams and seven people exploded into cascades of steam and debris this morning, and Lindy Schulz is dead. These are the watermarks of a person's life, lifetimes that find horse-drawn carriages giving way, giving way faster than anyone imagined, to the fireworks of liquid hydrogen.

Bruce Leonard is walking—slow shuffling steps, but even and steady. He has a goofy grin plastered on his face, his glasses slipped down to the end of his nose. He draws his right arm up to his chest, wrist turned inward, protective. Behind Bruce and Addie, who walks cautiously close beside him, is Bruce's father, shy, anxious, a little smile fixed on his face as he watches his son take—again—his first steps. He is scheduled to be transferred to a rehabilitation institute nearby, which specializes in head injuries. By tiny increments his personality is returning to flesh out the shell. "He was just an ordinary dude to begin with, so they don't expect him to be any more than that," says Nancy. The family has a strong religious faith, and privately Bruce's father tells Nancy it has helped them through a "terrible time which seems as though it has lasted for two years."

"He's trying to maintain control of his life," Paula tells a middle-aged woman who stands beside her near the nurses' desk. "It's *neat*. And we see this kind of thing all the time." Paula holds Jim Taub's chart as she talks, and when the woman leaves, Paula looks at Judy Currie, seated at the desk, and says, "*That* was a pack of lies."

Later in the morning Paula sits at her desk, smoking sensually. She relaxes in a joke, then spins to hunch over her desk and make a point, about Jim Taub and his gunshot wound, about head injury and brain damage and the clinical problems they entail. She is silent a moment, then points at the air in front of her and begins in a different voice.

"Thank God my daughter died." She waits a moment. "I'd often wondered, all these years of advising families, if I'd be able to have the same objectivity if it happened to me. And I was. I only had to take one look at her to know what the options were." She looks pointedly at the walls, beyond which are Buddy Mullin and Bruce Leonard and others. Lindy died in spite of the effort made, and Paula was spared too many choices. But her foreknowledge set her apart from her husband and the rest of Lindy's grieving relatives.

" 'How can you talk about her dying?' That's what they asked me. As though I *wanted* her to die. The doctor wouldn't even discuss organ donation with me, he was that freaked out.

"No one—*no one* talked to us about the possibility that she might die. The whole two days she lay in intensive care—*I* knew what was happening. And no one talked to us."

Paula might dismiss any notion of herself as innocent. She thinks, with a certain touch of pride, that her innocence disappeared a long time ago. But Paula was innocent of *this* pain, *this* loss, until New Year's Eve. It is her experience that tells her the loss is easier this way. She works now with a new understanding.

"If someone had just called me on the phone and said, 'Lindy's been killed,' I wouldn't have been able to make the kind of adjustment I've made. I wouldn't be here now. That little bit of time was so important."

Once a month Dr. Bob Strand, Harvest Moon's medical director, comes to the home for a luncheon meeting of the medical staff, which doubles as the Utilization Review Committee. In attendance are Paula and Janet; the pharmacist Ed Lewton, whose workmanlike sorting of papers and jars of pills is essential; Roger Scarpelli; and another physician, Dr. Matson, who has several patients at Harvest Moon.

Even while the members serve themselves from the buffet—the formica of the conference table covered for once with a tablecloth—Robert's Rules of Order are in effect. A curious formality pervades the conversation. Most of the people present see each other every day, and share a comfortable familiarity. But Drs. Strand and Matson aren't addressed by first names here, and humor and teasing directed toward them has a careful tone. They are meant to be pleased.

Dr. Strand is a dainty man, with poor posture; he hunches over his soup in a tailored, dark gray suit with a white linen shirt that looks freshly pressed. He is quiet, attentive, and talks rapidly and to the point. He takes the seat at the head of the table. Opposite him, Dr. Matson edges to a chair; she is eight months pregnant.

The Utilization Review Committee is mandated by Medicare for two purposes—to prepare studies of "patterns of care" and to determine "appropriate cost-effectiveness of care"—in other words, to decide whether individual patients qualify for Medicare coverage. Medicare analysts can override a URC decision, but the URC decisions are still required. Harvest Moon is expected to recruit and compensate, at least nominally, the members of the committee, which must include at least two physicians. The committee then meets at intervals determined by itself, and reviews individual cases as frequently as desired by the committee. When the URC turns thumbs down on a patient, and decides to revoke that patient's Medicare eligibility, it must say so in writing to the facility—Harvest Moon—the patient's physician, and the patient or his family, within two days. The payments stop seventy-two hours after the decision is made, not counting a day of discharge.

Paula Schulz coordinates the committee, preparing the cases to be presented and compiling required statistics, like the average length of stay. She is supposed to know at all times how long each Medicare patient's benefit period will last. Once she convinced the URC to continue a patient's benefits, then forgot how much more time they'd agreed to. But such gaps are rare in Paula's mind.

"I'm not allowed to bias the committee," she told me before the meeting. "I merely present the information." It is Paula's job to prepare the list, describe the patients up for review. Every Medicare patient comes up for review at least twice in a hundred-day period, and Paula is supposed to know which patients may be dangerously close to being ineligible for Medicare. "Nursing is allowed to try to bias the committee, and rehabilitation. If a patient is borderline, we usually decide ahead of time that we're going to let utilization review have them." It sounds suspiciously like holding off a wolf pack. And Paula does bias the committee, by her choice of words, her offhand comments, and her tone of voice, which ranges from pleading to an I-dare-you challenge.

Paula presents patients by a code number and description of their medical and nursing problems. Within this framework, between Robert's Rules of Order, soup, and salad, decisions are made quickly and with finality.

"You gave him the I.V.—because?" Dr. Strand questions Paula about her decision in a case. An I.V. alone might keep an otherwise stable patient on the skilled wing; Paula's reasoning is vital. Strand is Paula's supervisor, and the physician of record for a number of patients that are cared for on a daily basis by Paula.

"Because he's about ninety percent brain-dead," she snaps back, confusing the issue. Another patient, in a permanent coma, has been put on clysis, the technique of injecting fluids

177

through a needle directly into the muscle. It was done, says Paula, "because her daughter needed it."

Paula describes a new patient who appears to be failing to progress. She is blind, with a severe case of diabetes and a fractured hip. Her other leg was recently amputated below the knee because of complications from the diabetes, and today she has the flu.

"The question is whether or not she's skilled," points out Dr. Strand. "She's *sick,* but is she skilled?"

Paula argues that the woman's problems are complex and multiple, requiring the judgment and knowledge of a professional nurse. She says this with a touch of triumph.

"Is that a criterion?" asks Dr. Matson, her fork still. She looks at Dr. Strand. Paula explains that it can be.

"She sounds like a real challenge," says Strand. "You really need some sight in order to learn to balance on a prosthesis. Can she do it? If she can do it, she deserves a chance." The committee votes for continued coverage.

CHAPTER FOURTEEN

The Long Dream

I am leaning against a wall near the social worker's little office, watching a procession of wheelchairs cruise very slowly by. It is Valentine's Day, and a wave of shiny red hearts and lace trails down every hallway; there is one above my head. In the midst of the crowd leaving the dining room after lunch is a short, stout woman with the face of a bulldog. Her cheeks hang in jowls on both sides of an upper lip bristling with dark hair. She peers out from under her brow with small, bright eyes, rhythmically heaving her chair forward foot by foot. When she is opposite me, she stops, ponderously turns and gazes at me for a moment, up and down, and then speaks in a low, harsh voice.

"I don't have to talk to *you*," she says, her words authoritative, confident. "Who the hell do you think you *are*, anyway?" And then this woman, who has never spoken to me before, turns back to her task and continues on her way.

This is Maude Davis, ninety-three years old. She has lived in Harvest Moon for five years. Her reputation in this time has grown to mythic proportion—buoyed by streams of obscenities, unprovoked insults, slaps in the face that the staff has long ago learned to avoid. She is wily and sure of herself, thoroughly

179

disoriented about her surroundings, and seems sometimes to be spoiling for the entertainment of a good fight. She spends long periods ruminating—and napping—in her room, coming out only for meals and an occasional activity. It was she who knew Bobby Orr as the 1960 *Sports Illustrated* Sportsman of the Year. The affection she inspires in the staff is not wholly grudging; it is the affection lent to a horse that won't be broken. In her anger is a hot spark of life.

"I love her," says Margery Todd. "She's a delight. She's so—different."

Several times I have talked with Maude's daughter, Dorothy Krug, on the phone. She is loquacious about her mother, more than willing to discuss what she calls "the situation." But she invites me to her home to do so; in spite of her loyal visits to Harvest Moon every Wednesday morning, the place depresses her. She prefers her own immaculate house overlooking a golf course, carpeted in untouched white shag. When I arrive she pours me tea from a flowered pot that plays "Tea for Two" in chimes.

"Once a week we'd go shopping and have lunch," she remembers, "and we never went through the grocery store but that the clerk would look and say, 'This must be your daughter.' " She is proud of that fact, of the visible reminder of the closeness she has always felt to her mother. The daughter is slimmer, seasoned, with white hair in perfect, even waves. She moves fast and often, talks quickly, in whole paragraphs.

"I've just enjoyed my mother so much," she says cheerfully. "We just went everywhere together. She was always ready with a suitcase packed, always willing to do her share. A lot of fun. I don't think we ever missed a year that she wasn't with us for vacation.

"She never had any confidence in herself, so she liked to come across as though she didn't care whether she was with people or not. She always said she didn't *like* so-and-so. Well, it wasn't that she didn't *like* so-and-so, it was that she was afraid of so-and-so. She was always pretty independent, but this isn't independence," she says, referring to the hostility so apparent and uncontrolled now. "She's very angry. We had a chance to work into it gradually; otherwise, I think I would have been very nervous."

For years Maude Davis lived in a small, upstairs apartment down the street from Dorothy and her family. Dorothy was beginning to wonder how to approach her mother with the idea of moving to a retirement home when she fell and broke her hip. It was "perfect, in a way," says Dorothy now, because Maude could no longer argue against the move. It was a logical choice. But soon after she settled in, she had a heart attack, and Dorothy traces Maude's mental decline from there. Each year her confusion has increased, and spared Maude the knowledge of her own deterioration. She has never troubled Dorothy with complaints or pleas. And Dorothy in turn consoles herself, in the guilt she can't completely shake, that her mother wouldn't have wanted anything else.

"She always said, 'I *never* want to live with my kids!' She meant she didn't want to be a burden. We would have had to remodel, because there's no bedrooms on the first floor. And I could see far enough into the future to know it would not have been a happy situation for very long." Dorothy is resigned to her mother's life in an institution, and resigned to her own ambivalence about it, her own eternal wishes that it could be another way, a domestic fantasy. "I don't actually *know* anybody who's been happy with that situation. I think maybe it's kind of a fairy-tale thing that you read about, and you see how the grandmother is a kind of matriarch and the children and grandchildren are all happy, and everything is just geared around grandmother. I don't think it's fair when you have little children, and I think it's very unfair to a husband, usually. How can you be torn between a husband and your children and then your mother? It's hard enough to spread yourself around. People do it, bring their parents home, out of guilt, out of the terrible feeling that they *should* have done it, and then they resent it."

Even when the only realistic option is institutionalization, families hesitate to make the move. Studies, both private and government-sponsored, have shown that almost ninety percent of the care of frail elderly people is given by family members. Many of these people are victims of Alzheimer's disease and other dementias, and the relatives who provide home nursing may spend more than forty hours a week in direct care, up at night with a wanderer, sorting piles of soiled laundry, coaxing food down a reluctant eater. These are the tasks of a new and horrible parenthood. As a person's condition deteriorates, most families need to rely on outside help, which doesn't come cheaply. Placing a parent in a nursing home, though, is a kind of admission of failure, of being unable to support and carry the parent the way the parent carried the child decades before. The obvious differences—of age, and size, and inevitable decline—do little to salve that despair.

"My sister and I did just like you do—the hospital gave us a list and we just went around and visited several places. That was probably the hardest thing I'd ever done. We went to a couple of places that were supposed to be pretty nice, and we walked in and it was just, oh, no. So we were happy to find Harvest Moon.

"She's never fought anything, except going to therapy. Then she starts crying. But I think, my Lord, she's ninety-three years old! Why *should* she do anything she doesn't want to do? She's *tired*."

From the beginning of her stay at Harvest Moon, Maude has responded to men with an almost pleasant cooperation. She cooperates with the male aides even while refusing to look at the nurses.

"The one my mother was just ga-ga over, of course, was a Spanish man," says Dorothy. "Good-looking, of course. Any time there's a male to do things for her, that's much more acceptable. She likes men.

"There was a time a few years ago, when every thought I had before I went to sleep at night, and every thought I had when I woke up in the morning, was Mother and what her situation was. It hurts, it hurts a lot," she muses. "But it's gonna happen to everybody, one way or the other, sooner or later. When she's mean, I just think, 'That isn't my *mother*, for heaven's sake. *She* would never say anything like that to *me* and mean it!' "

The Krugs no longer bring Maude Davis home for visits, even on Christmas. She no longer notices the passing of time and holidays enough to feel left out of any attendant celebration. But such a choice traces a line of guilt that Dorothy Krug can't shake, and it is coupled with another made last year: the Krugs put Maude on welfare.

"The money is horrendous," says Dorothy. "We always subsidized her, two hundred and some dollars a month. My first feeling was, it's going to be the best we can possibly afford for her. So for five or six or seven years, what her little income didn't cover we took care of. And we thought it was quite a bit, but then when she had to go into the nursing home, that was even more. But we have to consider that *we're* getting older, too, and who knows what we'll need in ten years? We thought about welfare a lot before we did it. It's something that my age group and our generation was taught that you just *don't do,* and yet when you're put in the situation it seems a little more realistic. It bothers me the most because I know how it would bother Mother if she understood it."

Several months ago Maude Davis began having episodes of vaginal bleeding. Her physician wanted to have her brought to his office so he could do a complete exam. Dorothy was horrified by the idea, but not by its intimacy. Maude has severe arthritis in her hips, and the undignified position such an exam requires would have caused her terrible pain. Paula Schulz was able to get the same look by rolling Maude on her side, in her bed at the nursing home, and found a minor problem easily corrected. Dorothy, who professes great admiration for Paula, recalls, "And Paula said to the doc, 'Now what are you going to do if you find something bad? Perform a hysterectomy on a ninety-three-year-old lady? Now, *come on!*' "

Two years ago, Maude was rushed to the hospital when her heart began to fail. Without Dorothy's knowledge, a pacemaker was inserted in Maude's chest, a small device that triggers the heartbeat artificially, overriding its exhausted resignation. Pacemakers last for many years. When the doctors explained—after the fact—to Maude what they had done, she said, "No, I don't think so. I think I've been around long enough."

"At that time I thought, 'Now, doesn't that sound like Mother!' " recalls Dorothy. "As I look back, I think she really meant it. But who's to say? I wouldn't want to see her with all those tubes and the life support. No way." Dorothy pours more tea; the teapot sings. "She said to me something nasty the other day about someone being ninety-three, and I said, 'Well, *you're* ninety-three.' And she said, 'I think you should *croak* when you're ninety-three.' "

Dementia—most people call it senility—takes several forms. In the latest annual survey of nursing homes in the United States about half of all residents were institutionalized *primarily* because of some form of dementia. About half of all cases of permanent dementia are caused by Alzheimer's disease, a progressive destruction of essential brain tissues of unknown cause. Phoebe White has Alzheimer's disease. So does Cecil Lunt and Millie Peterson. Maude Davis probably has it, too, but like many elderly confused patients, her physician has not seen fit to diagnose it formally. The behavior of people with Alzheimer's is variable and unpredictable. Phoebe White slides into confusion with upright posture, her tears feminine and her tantrums minor and childish. Cecil Lunt has moved from precipitate, hot-headed motion into an abbreviation of motion itself. (Until she died last year, Cecil's wife lived down the hall from him at Harvest Moon, also an Alzheimer's victim. Her disease drove her to heights of comical gibberish, a wild-haired, skinny, incessantly talking woman who rarely made sense, likely to reach up as you walked by and grab your arm with long fingers ending in clawlike nails. There was nothing frightful about her; the jumble of meaning and her obvious frailty were a tender, even pathetic combination; not mad, but a parody of madness.)

Certain symptoms are common to Alzheimer's patients, and characterize the disease's course. The loss of memory and ability is gradual rather than sudden, and colored by an often incongruous talent at meaningless, trivial conversation—the stuff of brief daily encounters. This is what we ignobly preserve in our subconscious, patterned in our brain in a million places, through a lifetime of practice. Victims of the disease are often physically healthy, and remain so until the extremes of their demented behavior drive them into sickness—pneumonia from exposure, malnutrition, falls. The first thing lost is today, and the second thing tomorrow. Yesterday is held till last, but goes with time.

Some writers have characterized Alzheimer's patients as children, and the "second childhood" is a common expression. But it isn't their childishness that elicits the tenderness that I feel, and share with many people who come in contact with them. They reveal a naïveté and innocence that is, superficially, like childhood, but is built on the experiences of a lifetime. And children have a future, however immediate or distant it seems; Cecil and Phoebe and Maude go on and on and on into a future that they no longer conceive. I can't be in their presence and remain attached to any single purpose; their presence is the continual creation of the moment, such that any sentence begun has an ending that can't be predicted, any gesture a transient and irredeemable meaning. A face opens like an iris, and just as suddenly swirls shut. They give me a gift of non-Euclidean sight, until I dip and bend with the motion of a damaged cortex like a tree in wind. "Dreaming

185

was meant for nighttime," sang the Strumming Fool a month ago, as the white heads bobbed in rhythm. "I live in dreams all the day."

The logic is terpsichorean, but still logic; I believe that if I could somehow follow the neural sparks on their newly jogging paths, I would understand their direction, see the pattern—and that the pattern, however intricate or odd, would be made of the billion pieces of a long life held captive there: a sheet fluttering in a summer wind, its scent intoxicatingly wet and fresh; a window glimpsed high above the street by a child peering out the back seat of a car; sudden ripples of spring leaves under a full moon; a baby's cry, a baby's babble, and the downy skin; the crunch of fresh bread and the splash of wine on the white tablecloth underneath. "What could be sweeter than dreaming?" asks the singer. It is why they aren't children, and why I am made softer beside them, kinder; they are my elders.

The word *senility* carries with it the sense of inevitability; my *Webster's* defines it as "of or typical of old age." Not much is typical of old age, and certainly not senility; nor is there anything typical or predetermined about the skewed pathways dementia takes. I prefer the more technical word *dementia*, with its literary roots of mad kings and spiritual hallucination. It is the proper word, as Alzheimer's is properly called senile dementia of the Alzheimer's type, or SD:AT; just as the slate-clean destruction of strokes that leave people like Conrad Berry and Irma Washington helpless is properly called multi-infarct dementia, or MID. Both target in their arbitrary glee only a small percentage of the population. But like the relatively few deaths that occupy a disproportionate part of our concern, dementia is larger than its own life. Their victims are the forgotten children of social programs; they account for so many of the patients in nursing homes in part because these patients are frequently banned from retirement communities by diagnosis alone, regardless of their behavior.

At a care conference Paula is talking about Ruby, "one of

the grand old ladies of the place," who has been a patient for many years and now is declining into shadows. "There's a nephew who comes once a year and tries to make sure everyone knows he was here, and then he goes away for another year," she says, and imitates the expression of disgust Gina Tyrell reserves for him.

"You do a pretty good Gina," Nancy compliments her. "Ruby needs reassurance on *everything*—is she going to dinner on time, is she dressed properly, everything."

"She told a Catholic priest I beat her up," adds Margery Todd. "She wanted her driver's license back yesterday."

"Did you give it to her? Did you offer to loan her your car?" asks Paula.

"I kind of hedged on it," Margery answers.

It is typical to speak about such behavior, so common, so tenderly amusing, as "undignified," to assume that if the person knew their actions they would feel degraded somehow, humiliated. It is a moot point, of course, in every sense of the word—the point is that they don't know, and can't. Yet a kind of logic persists: How many times have I been accosted by a person restrained in a wheelchair who asked, politely, if I had scissors with which to cut the annoying strap? Nancy Rice tells me about a woman who had to be fed separately from other patients because of her habits, which she cherished: "She would put all her condiments—her honey and salt and sugar and all—on her eggs, and eat her Rice Krispies with a fork." I am reminded of a woman from long-ago aide work, a demon when crossed, who settled happily into any meal—pancakes, lamb chops, chocolate cake—as long as it was smothered in ketchup. People hide in closets, hitch rides. I know of a patient who left her nursing home, flagged down a car, and told the male driver she'd been at a party where people were "smoking and drinking," that she'd grown disgusted and needed a ride to the nearest shopping center. He believed her. By the time she was found, with the help of the police, she'd forgotten the whole thing and was happy to be "home." Nurses take a black amusement in such stories—what else could they take from them? The only alternative is a blacker grief, or despair at the pathetic turns life leads us on. Erin Myers says, "They provide moments of lighter humor, which aren't in great abundance." Why should something over which a person has no control be shameful? Why should the sweet, skewed wisdoms of Alzheimer's be more embarrassing than paralyzed legs or deaf ears—as the latter used to be? It isn't really a judgment of right and wrong, but one of pity, and pity is the great creator of distance. How can anyone *lose* their dignity? They are still—tied in wheelchairs, outlandish, incongruous—my elders.

"We don't believe in restraining patients," says Janet Krause. "*I hate it*. I hate seeing them in a wheelchair when they are perfectly capable of walking around. But if we can't provide a safe environment, that's our alternative." (A lot of staff, not to mention families and visitors, hate seeing restraints. But many staff refuse to feel any apology for them, knowing the alternative is usually injury. At one care conference Paula was bemoaning a particular patient's fate. "It's pathetic to see her restrained," she said. Charlene Parrott just snorted. "I think we should *chain* her to her wheelchair," she answered.) "For the minimum time," Janet continues, "we use restraints with walking periods during the day. And meanwhile we look for another placement, a safer place that could provide for them with the physical needs they have."

The safer place, now and in the future, may be a special care unit, or SCU, a new concept being enthusiastically tried at many nursing homes across the country. SCUs are specifically for demented patients in relatively good health, like Phoebe White and Gertrude Werner. They are wide, specially designed wings with locked doors (usually secured by electronic code locks that automatically unlock when the fire alarm is activated) and separate exercise and activity areas. Part of the point of an SCU is the avoidance of restraint, and patients are often allowed to wander the halls and in and out of each other's rooms. Because they are all demented, this intrusion causes little dismay. The staff is carefully selected and specially trained, and the turnover in such units, so far, is lower than average. There is less physical care, less exhaustion, fewer medications—and no chasing or fear of lost patients. When I visited an SCU near my home, the twenty-some residents sat in a horseshoe near a small organ, while a woman played ragtime. A few beat their chair arms, several slept, one man walked forward and backward methodically over the same few feet. A little woman sidled up to me silently, and began fingering the cardigan sweater I wore over my shirt. I put my arm around her shoulder—she was no taller than my nine-year-old son—and she huddled up close. "Are you cold?" I asked her. "Do you want a sweater, too?" And she looked at me with great relief, expression opening her face bright and wide with light, and nodded yes, yes.

For years dementia was attacked with the good intentions of therapeutic theory; nurses were trained to use "reality orientation," a constant, nagging tug back to the present place and time. RO, as it's called, was a classic lesson in frustration with the demented. It works, sometimes, for psychiatric patients, for people whose confusion stems from the environment, as in intensive care units. With people whose brains can no longer retain information, who literally can't *learn*, it fails miserably.

"I've seen reality orientation really agitate patients," says Janet. " 'It isn't 1943, it's 1986.' They *want* to be in 1943. Who are you to say where those forty years went, and who are you to say I'm not who I think I am? Instead, 'It's 1943, how nice. And what are we doing right now?' And in a few moments they forget."

The other failed solution with dementia is medication—sedatives and tranquilizers, used to attempt control of wandering, aggression, even depression—or what *appeared* to be depression. "A lot of the time they get overmedicated," Janet says. "I have a real problem with that, to see someone who's alive and walking and *not* in 1986, but *walking,* feeding themselves and dressing themselves, become a person who is a zombie. We try everything before we look at medication."

Few demented patients need skilled nursing care, and dementia alone is no criterion for it. And oh, what little hope there is for rehabilitation! So Medicare will cover none of the costs specific to the dementia. (If an Alzheimer's patient gets pneumonia or breaks a hip—*and* they are over sixty-five, which many are not—then Medicare will cover the costs of that illness or accident as usual. But when the benefit period is over or the illness is cured, benefits stop.) There is talk now and then of "entitling" Alzheimer's disease the way kidney disease was entitled years ago—making a specific provision in the Medicare law to cover the costs of that disease. But Alzheimer's disease can only be definitively diagnosed after death, by autopsy, and diagnosis until then is an empirical work of experience. With entitlement would come a flood of Alzheimer's diagnoses, a veritable epidemic.

A few days ago Phoebe White was reviewed at care conference. Nancy Rice noted that she was doing less for herself, crying more often.

"She likes having things done for her," said Paula.

"Well, most of the time Phoebe's happy, so that's all right," said Margery.

"She can really work herself into some kind of physical illness with worry," Paula added, noting that her money was almost gone and her son, who had recently moved from another city to be near her, was planning to apply for welfare for her care.

"We could lie to her," said Margery.

"She responds well to lies," said Nancy.

" 'Lie to patient and reassure her,' " Paula answered, pretending to write in the case note.

" 'And tie her hands down when she won't take her medication and make her take it so she won't get sick!' " called out Nancy, in an atmosphere suddenly giddy.

" 'Lie and tie up!' " quoted Paula.

" 'Lie and abuse!' " murmured Charlene Parrott.

Meeting for lunch today is a group nearly identical to the group that met for utilization review a few weeks earlier: Paula, Janet, Roger, Nancy, and Drs. Strand and Matson are joined by Edie Douglas, the administrative assistant, for soup and salad, small triangular ham sandwiches, and lemon pudding. The menu in the dining room is slightly different; before the door is shut a loud, cheery voice can be heard asking, "Ya wanna hot dog?"

This group meets as the ethics committee, set up to discuss policy and make recommendations to the medical staff meeting. Today the discussion centers on the need for a written consent form from families before a do not resuscitate (DNR) order is adopted for a patient. Paula opens the talk by describing how she solved that problem with Herbert Kincaid, a childless widower with Alzheimer's disease whose only relative is a mentally ill sister in another state. Kinkaid's health is rapidly failing, and he seems at risk for a heart attack soon. So Paula called the sister, who immediately agreed to a DNR without knowing its purpose.

"You called the *sister?*" says Edie, a little shocked.

"Well, what would *you* do?" retorts Paula. "Code Herbie Kincaid? Not *this* kid."

After thirty minutes of amiable discussion and mild disagreement on responsibility, a form is approved. The only difficulty is determining the line of responsibility within a family. If there is no spouse, who is next empowered to decide? Siblings or children—or, in some cases, parents? Edie dismisses the problem, saying "Just be sensible," to deal with each case individually. "We know best who to ask for each patient," she adds.

191

The form is to be forwarded to the medical staff meeting, but Dr. Strand points out that such a quorum of the medical staff committee is at the table right now. He convenes the committee and calls for a vote. The form is approved, the committee is adjourned, and the ethics committee reconvenes for further conversation.

In getting the form approved, Paula suggests they begin with intermediate-care patients: "the walking-talking-smoking-screaming-at-staff patients," she says. "It won't be a problem. Families don't expect us to code patients in a nursing home."

Nancy wants the forms filled out within three months, and Paula looks at her witheringly. "I've been working on this for *six years,* and all of a sudden you want it in a few weeks!"

Dr. Matson, still pregnant, has been silent, but Paula's remark stirs her. Another nursing home where she has patients decided to call every patient's physician and get DNR orders in just two days. There was no contact with families. She shakes her head. "Even now, they'll call me about patients I'll be picking up when they leave the hospital and ask me for a no-code order before I've even met them."

Edie Douglas has been trying to determine how frequently physicians must visit their patients; there is disagreement between state and Medicare and facility regulations. She picks delicately at a piece of lettuce in her bowl, then wipes her hand on her napkin before explaining that when she called the state, the answer was a visit every 120 days.

"I broke the cardinal rule—never ask a bureaucrat after you've identified yourself," she smiles. "I fully expect that in a hundred twenty days they'll be breathing down our necks to make sure our visits are up-to-date."

But it isn't always easy to get a physician to visit. Dr. Matson says she knows doctors who will charge a patient for an ambulance call to bring them to the doctor's office for a routine checkup rather than visit a dreaded nursing home. "Some of them are only five blocks away. It's shameful."

There is another point, too. If a patient is covered by Medicare, there is no guarantee that Medicare will pay even a portion of the cost of that ambulance. For the doctor's convenience, a patient or his family may be billed for the costly—and unnecessary—service.

"It *is* changing, though," says Roger. "Ten years ago we never could have gotten even one physician, let alone two, to sit down and dialogue with us like this."

As the meeting breaks up, with the scraping of chairs and the careful, polite shuffling of several people in a cramped space, someone wonders out loud if the ethics committee is really useful, if perhaps the makeup and purpose of the committee shouldn't be reconsidered. After a few moments of casual discussion, Edie Douglas's voice rises over the quiet murmurs. "Well, we need *some*thing," she says, almost apologetically. "There have got to be ethical issues we deal with, oh, every hour or so."

CHAPTER FIFTEEN

Shine On, Shine On

It is a beautiful and perfectly clear day, a day of short sleeves and no clouds. The trees and bushes are suddenly draped in pink and ivory, the air thick with the smell of the mock-orange hedge in front of Harvest Moon. The bare lacy limbs have lines of nubbins along their branches like borders of crochet. Inside it is harder to see evidence of the earth's gradual tilt. There is a vase of daffodils on the file cabinet, but the fluorescent light is the same as that of November or July.

Many things are the same as they were in November and last July—and will remain the same through another July, and another. The shifts are subtle ones, the dance mild and slow, chastening, wavelike. I will never be as taut as I once was, or as smooth—I am several months older now than last October, just like Phoebe and Max. My breasts are already beginning their long sag, my hips their white lines; I have small, premonitory wrinkles in the corners of my eyes. I see the fine, lilac map, barely visible, of my mother's and grandmother's varicose veins on the inside of my calf. Things happen to each of us, and they leave indelible, nearly transparent marks that pile gradually, year by year, atop each other till their presence is unmistakable. And my grandmother is dead, and my mother dying—and my turn comes soon, too soon.

Roles blur; I am one moment nurse, authority; another moment daughter, and full of fear. I walk the halls of Harvest Moon, feeling them lap at my heels, curve around me. I'm home here, and I can't go away. I have been in and out of Harvest Moon, and several other nursing homes, off and on for years. This time I came to Harvest Moon just to watch, to see what I could see. Nursing homes are hard places, and they make complex demands of overlapping and conflicting purpose; my observations overlap with my experience, and my ignorance. The familiarity I find so comfortable is laced with a ligature of eccentricity. Standing still in the midst of such clockwork pandemonium, I see a wee movement, a quiet caress, fraternal and weary, and it is like a real and heroic act winning out by endurance over great and constant odds.

This community remains much the same. It is an interactive society of fluid dependencies and small gratifications, no more linear than the conversation of my demented friends—but fluctuating, spiral, helical by nature. I come over and over to the same viewpoint from different heights, always moving, never still. That's what the old have taught me, and the weak: past, future, present, like many mountaintops in a range. These vistas pass so quickly, quickly by, glimpses caught in half my eye, grasped after and gone.

At eleven in the morning two women arrive and walk promptly to the dining room, where one sits at the battered piano without a word and begins to play a line of melody over and over. The other woman, dressed in a navy skirt and blazer with the short gray hair of a prison matron, sorts a file full of notes. It is time for church, which Judy Currie forgot to announce, and for fifteen minutes the aides hunt for interested participants, finding at last seven: six white-haired women, all in wheelchairs, and Max Kleiner, parked discreetly several yards away. Margaret Bond and two others silently share the

Sunday newspaper at the smokers' table. Every few minutes, as the lunch hour approaches, an aide will come through the hissing double doors and clank change into the vending machines.

The piano swells slightly into a verse, sung without preliminary by the gray-haired woman. Her voice is high and rings in the big, empty room.

"I need thee every hour, most gracious Lord," she sings, full of feeling. "I need Thee, oh, I need Thee! Every hour I need Thee!" Her audience is sitting in a semicircle in front of her, and as she sings she passes out big-print hymnals bound inside manila folders.

"We thank you, Father, for enabling us to be here today," she intones at the end of her song. "Thank you for the staff people who have helped us to be here. Oh, Father, we ask you to give us a special lift in the coming week, encouragement in our physical frailties, and spiritual strength. In Jesus Christ's name, amen." At the end of the prayer she looks at her clasped hands, then abruptly raises her head, her manner and tone changed.

She speaks then of King David, and how he prayed in the fields while tending sheep. "He had the whole sky to see, to admire the handiwork of God," she says, sweeping her hand across the air in front of her. "David was a man after God's own heart. Are *we* people after God's own heart?" She looks searchingly at the horseshoe in front of her. The pianist waits respectfully, slightly behind the minister. "God's love is unconditional. He forgives us. We have trouble forgiving ourselves."

At eleven thirty the smoking aide arrives with a wicker basket full of cigarette packages. She sorts the packs, hands each person at the smokers' table a cigarette, and lights them, one after the other.

"Yea, Thou art my rock and my fortress; for Thy name's sake lead me and guide me," she reads from Psalm 31, one of David's Psalms. "I am the scorn of my adversaries, a horror to my neighbors, an object of dread to my acquaintances; those who see me in the street flee from me. I have passed out of mind like one who is dead; I have become a broken vessel."

She gazes first at her Bible, in silence, then at the faces before her, as though suddenly realizing the implication of the verse she chose. "Consider it pure joy," she finishes, smiling, "pure *joy* whenever you face trials of many kinds." She nods to the pianist. "We'll sing number eleven, 'Draw Me Nearer, O Lord.'"

After lunch the dining room clears and two long tables are pulled together. Margery Todd, a little flustered, checks the positions of chairs, clears a space for wheelchairs. The big console radio near the smokers' table plays hard rock, "American Woman," raucous and loud.

Once a month the resident council meets here, to discuss problems with staff, ideas for new activities. It is a loosely organized panel with no membership requirements other than that of residence. In the last few meetings, a number of people expressed unhappiness about the nursing staff, and today Janet Krause is scheduled to come to the council and answer questions.

Tillie Mott is wheeled to a place beside Buddy Mullin, who sits tall and straight in his padded, high-backed chair.

"Three Questions and Bingo?" she says brightly to the table of faces around her.

"No, did someone promise you that?" asks Margery.

"Yes! What is it?" replies Tillie with concern.

"It's resident council."

"Never heard of it," humphs Tillie, dropping her chin to her chest.

Phoebe White finds a place near a corner of the table, and points a long, bony finger at Margery.

"Are you the boss? Are you the boss?" she demands.

"Lambikins, this is resident council," Margery patiently answers.

"They *said* they'd take me for a walk," complains a stout woman seated nearby. Phoebe turns to her.

"You're a big shot," she says with scorn.

Robert Zittle whirs into the room, his heavy electric chair swift and firm among the hesitant self-starters. He honks the horn attached to one armrest, and half the sleepy women jump. He smiles the one-sided smile allowed by his illness, and chuckles.

"We'll go ahead and start," calls out Margery. "Can everyone hear me? Welcome to resident council. We usually go around at the beginning and introduce ourselves. I'm Margery Todd, the activity director."

One by one the names are spoken, in various voices. Buddy names himself with staccato brevity and turns to look at Tillie Mott, staring into her lap.

"Introduce yourself," he says to her gruffly.

"What?"

"We're introducing ourselves," he says again.

"*You* didn't introduce yourself," she replies, petulant.

"Buddy Mullin," he says, with reproach in his voice now.

"What?"

"Buddy Mullin!"

"Buddy Mullin?"

"*Yes!*"

"Oh," she answers, mollified. "Well, I'm Tillie Mott."

Max Kleiner watches eagerly from outside the circle. He wears an enormous green and white Hawaiian shirt. Margery reads the minutes of the last meeting, and asks, "How are things going with the call lights?"

Robert Zittle slowly raises his hand. He is heavy, like his chair, curled forward on his own round stomach like a ball; he must look up from under his thick brows in order to see the group. He wears a maroon polyester suit, his best clothes, reserved for church and family holidays and business. He talks in a slow, stilted whisper with breathy pauses.

"About the call light," he begins. "I have a. Tough time. Getting anyone. To answer. An hour. Two hours and ten min-

198

utes," he says, holding up his hand for emphasis. "Is a long time. You'd be dead. Before they came."

Margery looks worried. "Sounds like it's still a problem. Let's wait till Janet's here. She should be here any time." She glances at the clock. Janet is fifteen minutes late.

Margery talks about the new Bible study class and different activities scheduled for the coming month, and after another five minutes Janet Krause hurries into the room.

Margery introduces her, finishing, "She's available just to answer your questions."

"Hello," says Janet, then glances back to Margery. "Do they have any questions?"

"Call lights," says Robert Zittle. "They're not. Getting answered."

"Is that a problem for everyone?" asks Janet, frowning.

"Two hours. Too long," adds Robert.

"What?"

"Two *hours*. Too long," he repeats, a little smile on his face.

"Well, I'm not sure why this is a problem," answered Janet. She promises to talk to the administration, then get back to Margery with a response.

"This may be silly, but why do bedpans have to be out of sight at nighttime?" asks Elizabeth Grove, seated across from Buddy. "I can't reach it. I have a pad, but I don't care to wet it." She holds her flaccid arm gently in her lap.

"It's just one of those things nurses are taught, about cleanliness, aesthetics, germ control. If you have a special request we can work with that." She turns away, but Elizabeth isn't through.

"Then there's the noise in the hall at night," she adds.

"Oh, it's terrible, four o'clock in the morning," adds another voice, and there is general murmuring agreement around the table.

"I need to tell you that at night the noises amplify. It probably sounds a lot louder than it is," Janet answers. "I can talk to staff."

"I hear them going down the hall laughing, and I don't know what they're laughing about!" says a woman at the end of the table.

"I say 'Shut up out there!' " says Sophie Feldman.

"Yes, I know you do," replies Margery.

"It works, too," adds Sophie.

"I do, too," says Buddy. "I say shut up."

Margery leans over the table. "I think we need to say nice things to each other. Let's talk about nice things. What *good* things have happened to people lately? Let's talk about the good aides."

"There's darn few," Robert says again.

Elizabeth Grove speaks again. She holds herself with dignity, on a determined course. "We've got this little box with a door and drawer by our bed, to put all our worldly goods in. And if we put money in it, it's gone in one night. I don't have any money around me any more. And the other day this girl came in and threw away a bunch of stuff. Those are my things in that damned box. And she didn't even ask."

"Well, that's not right," replies Janet. "They have to have your permission. That's true for all of you."

"Bugging me," says Buddy. "Howie is bugging me. At night. Ticks me off."

"You have to talk to Nancy Rice about that," answers Janet.

"I *did*."

"Maybe you and Nancy and I could sit down and talk about it."

She turns to go. "Do you all know where my office is? It's right by the nurses' desk. If you have any questions just come by and ask me."

"How many nurses are here at night?" asks Elizabeth. "Do they go home after they're done putting people to bed?"

"No, they stay here all night," replies Janet, and thanks the group for asking her to come.

"Come every time," says Robert Zittle.

"Every time?" she asks. "Well, it's always nice to see your smiling faces." She nods and leaves.

Margery turns to Elizabeth. "Lizzy, what wonderful thing has happened to you this week?"

"*Wonderful?* Nothing. Ha," says Elizabeth.

Sophie Feldman complains about a woman screaming at night. "I think someone's crazy down there. They just go on and on and keep me awake."

"How about you, Buddy? Anything wonderful?" Margery asks with determined cheer.

"Nope."

"Buddy is working hard in our ceramics program," Margery tells the council. "If any of you want to help, we could sure use you."

"Well, I'll tell you," says a small, white-haired woman. "We all have to do all we can for humanity. We're not alone. And that's my speech."

"*Well,* I'm glad you're feeling so positive!" beams Margery.

"I'm not doing so much," says a big man near Max. "I can't hear very well. I'm just setting."

"How are you, Ella?" Margery asks the woman beside her.

"I want to go back to my room," says Ella.

"In just a few minutes."

"I have to go to therapy, too," adds Ella.

"How are you, Max?"

"Wee-wee-wee! Bay-bay-bay," says Max. "Wah-wah."

"You're fine. Good," replies Margery. "Anybody else? Well, thanks for coming. See you next month."

Author's Note on Sources

For census and population statistics I relied on the National Nursing Home Survey of 1977 and the National Master Facility Inventory Survey Overview, both publications of the U.S. Department of Health and Human Services.

Specifics of Medicare and Medicaid coverage and related statistics are from *The Medicare and Medicaid Book* of 1981 and *Your Medicare Handbook,* both publications of the U.S. Department of Health and Human Services; the Office of Technology Assessment's report, *Medicare's Prospective Payment System: Strategies for Evaluating Cost, Quality, and Medical Technology;* and a number of conversations with administration and field personnel in the Health Care Financing Administration system.

Details of the diagnosis and rehabilitation of strokes are based on information in *Diagnosis and Management of Strokes and TIAs,* edited by John Stirling Meyer and Terry Shaw (Menlo Park, Calif.: Addison-Wesley, 1982) and *A Problem-Oriented Approach to Stroke Rehabilitation* by John W. Sharpless (2nd ed.; Springfield, Ill.: Charles C. Thomas, 1982), and numerous articles in the medical and nursing literature.

The following books provided a general profile of the theories and problems in long-term care, as well as substantiating statistics: *Health Care and the Elderly* by C. Carl Pegels (Rockville, Md.: Aspen Systems Co., 1980), *Last Home for the Aged: Critical Implications of Institutionalization* by Sheldon S. Tobin and Morton A. Lieberman (San Francisco: Jossey-Bass, 1976), *The Growth of Nursing Home Care* by Burton David Dunlop (Lexington, Mass.: Lexington Books, 1979), *Long Term Care of the Elderly: Public Policy Issues* by Charlene Harrington, Robert J. Newcomer, Carroll L. Estes, and Associates (Beverly Hills, Calif.: SAGE Publications, 1985), and "Crisis in Long-Term Care," parts I and II, by Charlene Harrington in *Nursing Economics* (Jan.–Feb. and Mar.–Apr. 1985, *3*, 15–20 and 109–115).

The article cited in Chapter 10 is "Turbulent Seas Stirred by DRGs," by Jerry L. Rhoads, *Nursing Homes* (Jan.–Feb. 1985).